Speaking of:
Diabetes

by Rüdiger Petzoldt, M.D.

Introduction by Karl Schöffling, M.D., Professor of Medicine

Translated by
Françoise E. Heyden

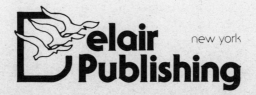

elair Publishing   new york

Rüdiger Petzoldt, M.D.
Born in 1938 in Wuppertal, Ruediger Petzoldt studied medicine in Marburg, Vienna and Frankfurt. He specialized in internal medicine in Ulm and Frankfurt. Dr. Petzoldt is presently chief resident in endocrinology and metabolism at the Center for Internal Medicine at the University of Frankfurt and a member of German and international medical societies. He has written numerous articles about diabetes for both physicians and patients.

Karl Schöffling, M.D., Professor of Medicine.
Born in 1921 in Sobernheim, Karl Schoeffling studied medicine in Heidelberg and Frankfurt. He is medical director of the Center for Internal Medicine and Head of the Department of Endocrinology and Metabolism at the University of Frankfurt. He is involved in research at American, Canadian and German Universities (Baltimore, Toronto, Frankfurt, Ulm) and is a member of German and international medical societies. He is the author of numerous articles and books.

Library of Congress Catalog Card Number: 80-68763
ISBN: 0-8326-2243-5

Originally published in German under the title *Sprechstunde: Diabetes*, copyright © 1979 by Gräfe und Unzer Verlag, München.

Contents

The Diabetic — Specialist in His Own Disease

Diabetes mellitus is one of the most frequent and common diseases of our time. At least 3% of the population in industrial nations is afflicted by this disease, 9 million persons in the U.S. alone. This figure is constantly on the rise and is actually higher when the unrecognized and therefore untreated diabetics are taken into consideration. It is estimated that about 1% of the population has untreated diabetes.

In addition, about 10% of the population, 22 million persons in the U.S., suffer from latent diabetes which can be discovered only through special medical tests. In this early stage diabetes does not cause symptoms, but it may develop into full diabetes later. Moreover, research has shown that a considerable number of perfectly healthy persons are genetically predisposed to develop the disease. These hereditary factors cannot be directly detected and occur in about 25% of the population. The incidence of diabetes and certain metabolic and other diseases has increased to nearly epidemic proportions.

every fourth is endangered

These other diseases include disorders of the fat metabolism, gout, and hypertension. They are "diseases of civilization" and are caused primarily by obesity, the wrong type of food intake and lack of exercise. They are the typical consequences of an oversupply of the three S's (starches, salt and sugar as well as fat) in industrialized nations. For each of these potentially harmful diseases and for diabetes in particular, good effective methods of treatment have been developed; in fact hardly any disease is cured as easily as diabetes when detected in the early stage. If however, the diabetic goes untreated or is only partially or improperly treated, then he incurs a much higher risk. Complications arising from diabetes, such as vascular damage leading to heart attack or stroke, pose a great danger to the improperly and untreated diabetic in particular. The effectiveness of the therapy can be measured by the decrease of the risk-factors and their sequelae.

4

It has been possible to treat all forms of diabetes successfully ever since Dr. F.G. Banting and the medical student C.H. Best applied a pancreatic extract to lower the elevated blood sugar of a diabetic dog. This experiment was performed on August 6, 1921 in Toronto and involved the removal of the dog's pancreas to induce diabetes. After insulin was discovered, it was continuously improved and further refined. Today the treatment of diabetes is based on methods developed earlier, as well as on the latest results of research. A properly balanced diet, effective medication and reasonable exercise will help to bring blood sugar under control and to avoid sugar in the urine. If the treatment is good and initiated in the early stage of disease, then the diabetic will be able to lead a nearly normal, happy and productive life. More than in any other disease, successful treatment of diabetes depends primarily on cooperation between the physician and the patient and on the specialization of the patient in his own disease, giving him the tools to treat himself successfully.

goal: normal-
ization of
metabolic
disorder

Physicians, dieticians and patients have collaborated in developing this book, even if they did not engage in the actual task of writing. All the topics discussed in this book were brought up many times in our medical consultations.

answers to
patients'
questions

We hope to answer as many of your questions as possible in this book. You can adopt the proper measures of treatment in order to stay active and to avoid harmful complications only if you know the answers to your questions. If you know how to treat diabetes successfully and if you use this knowledge in everyday situations, then you will attain the goals of diabetes therapy — as a specialist in your own disease.

Karl Schöffling

1. Diabetes, a Metabolic Disorder

Diabetes, or *diabetes mellitus* as it is called in medical terminology, has been known to doctors for more than three thousand years. One of the major signs of the disease, the increased frequency of urination, is already mentioned in the papyrus manuscripts written about 1500 B.C. Greek physicians first used the term "diabetes mellitus". "Diabetes" describes the increased urination and "mellitus" suggests the honey-like taste of the urine.

cause: insulin deficiency

But it was not until about 100 years ago that more was known about the nature of diabetes. Today we know that diabetes is caused by a lack of insulin. If the pancreas ceases to produce this hormone altogether, then the diabetic must take insulin for the rest of his life. (A *hormone* is a chemical substance formed in a gland of the body and transported by the blood stream.) In the case of relative insulin deficiency, an insufficient amount of insulin is secreted by the pancreas or is produced at the wrong time. Patients with this most frequent type of diabetes can usually be treated simply by an appropriate diet or by a diet combined with oral hypoglycemic agents.

Normal Sugar Metabolism

Diabetes is a disorder of metabolism. Before the disorder can be understood, the normal function of metabolism must be understood.

The food we consume is transformed by the digestive system to allow the organs to utilize it. The estimated 1000 billion cells composing the body are nourished by this food.

the digestive process

Cells can be seen only under a microscope and they can utilize food only when it is broken down into its elements. This breakdown of food starts with the process of eating, chewing and digesting in the mouth, stomach and intestines. Only the digestible parts of food can pass through the walls of the intestines into the blood stream. The cell needs these building

6

blocks to grow, to maintain itself, and to produce energy. The indigestible food components are excreted as bulk material with the bowel movement.

Our food intake consists of different parts which vary in quantity and in composition. Carbohydrates, fats and proteins are the three most important nutritive elements and are separated in the process of digestion. Carbohydrates include sugar and starches, and fats are also called lipids.

Our bodies need energy to maintain vital functions. The energy contained in carbohydrates, fats and protein (and thus in all food) can be measured. The term "calorie" has been used for a long time. (In physics the *calorie* is defined as the amount of heat needed to raise the temperature of one milliliter of water by one degree Centigrade from 14.5 degrees to 15.5 degrees.) A recent international agreement made the use of "joule" acceptable as a measure of energy value in foods, but "calorie" is used in the U.S.

Fats contain a large amount of energy: 1 gram of pure fat equals 9.3 calories (cal.). The fats are transported to the different organs via the blood stream, where they are either used up immediately or else stored for later use in fatty tissues. Proteins and carbohydrates contain less energy: 1 gram of protein or carbohydrate contains 4.1 calories.

Proteins are more of a source of building-blocks than a source of energy. Building blocks are indispensible for the body's own production of the protein that it must have. Proteins are the raw material for the production of cell substance, plasma protein, enzymes and hormones. (*Enzymes* are proteins created by the cell which make metabolism possible by acting like catalysts and causing, accelerating, or directing chemical reactions.)

Carbohydrates are the third major component of food and are found mainly in starches and sugar. Cane sugar is the common household sugar. Flour and flour products, rice, semolina, potatoes are a few examples of starches. During digestion, starches and sugar are turned into glucose (dextrose) and fructose, which are both called simple sugars.

Before we can understand the metabolic disorder of the diabetic, we must become familiar with the metabolism of a healthy person. The accompanying drawing will help us imagine the system which normally regulates blood sugar.

7

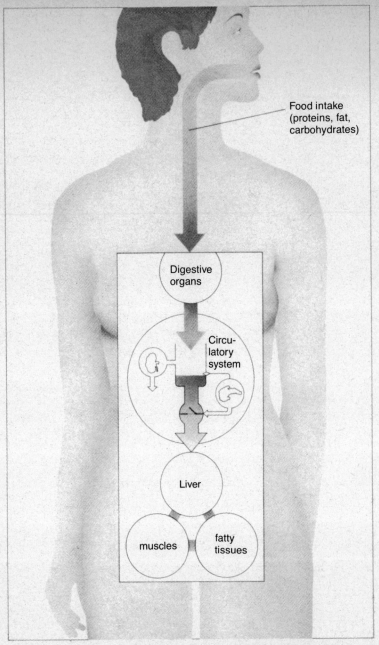

Food intake
(proteins, fat,
carbohydrates)

Digestive
organs

Circu-
latory
system

Liver

muscles

fatty
tissues

Digestion and metabolism: The break-down of food begins with the process of eating and digesting in the mouth, stomach and intestines. Digested nutritive elements pass through the intestinal wall into the blood stream. Insulin helps sugar flow into the liver, muscles and fatty tissues, where it is transformed and stored.

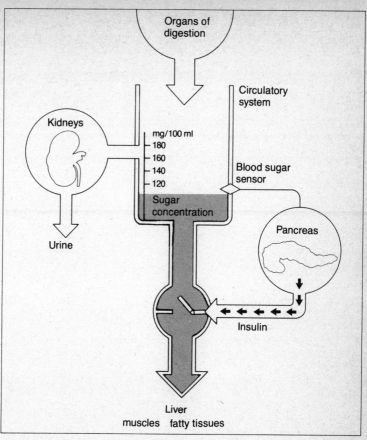

Normal sugar metabolism. Food intake causes the blood sugar concentration to rise. This causes the pancreas to secrete insulin. Insulin helps the sugar flow from the blood into the liver, muscles and fatty tissues where it serves as a source of energy or else is stored. In a normally functioning metabolism, the increased concentration of blood sugar remains at a normal low level and never reaches the renal threshold.

The carbohydrates in the food flow into a big pot which represents the total circulatory system. The concentration of blood sugar, which is always present in the blood, is fairly stable. The intake of carboydrates causes the blood sugar to rise temporarily within certain limits. The amount of sugar in the blood is measured in milligrams/100 milliliters (mg/100ml). The fasting value of blood sugar concentration in a healthy person is usually below 100 mg/ml (see table on normal values).

Insulin helps the sugar flow from the blood into the tissues and

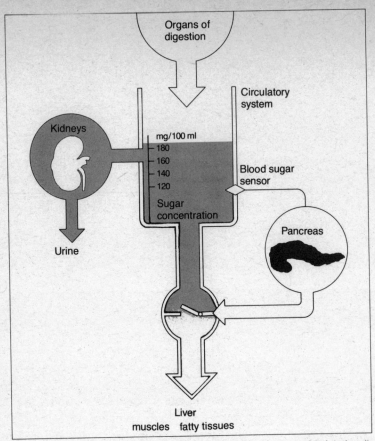

Abnormal sugar metabolism. The diabetic suffers either from an absolute insulin deficiency or from the inability of the pancreas to produce sufficient amounts of insulin. This absolute insulin deficiency and insufficiency of insulin disrupt the "regulatory mechanism" which normally causes the blood sugar to flow into the organs. As a result, the concentration of blood sugar is increased and surpasses the renal threshold. Sugar is then excreted in the urine and cannot serve as a source of energy for the system.

cells (a detailed explanation will be given later). The muscles are the first to utilize this sugar. They use the amount of glucose they need to facilitate movements. When the muscle is resting and does not need the sugar offered, the glucose is stored in other organs as an energy reserve.

The first storage place is the liver, the most important chemical factory of our body. Most of the break-down and build-up processes involved in food utilization occur in this organ. The glucose flowing into the liver via the blood stream is stored here

muscle nourishment from blood sugar

glycogen = reserve sugar

10

as so-called glycogen. The liver can store only a certain amount of glycogen, about 70 to 80 grams.

What happens to the sugar for which there is no storage room in the liver? The answers to these questions will explain the causes of obesity and the increase of fatty tissues.

excess car-
bohydrates
become fat

The excess carbohydrates can be converted into fat and stored in almost unlimited quantities in the fatty tissues. The same holds true for other food components which are not used as a source of energy or metabolized. As a result, everything we eat in excess is stored as fat and leads to obesity.

The Significance of Insulin

Which mechanism is responsible for the proper utilization of glucose and for keeping the blood sugar concentration at a normal level? How is this system regulated? The most important role is played by insulin. Its function is perhaps best explained by analogy with a thermostat in a central heating system using oil.

The upper value of the room temperature we wish to attain is 70°F, the lower value is 63°F (17°C); the heating system has been programmed for these two values. The thermostat measures the room temperature. When it rises above the upper value of 70°F (23°C), an electrical contact causes the heating system to be turned off. Similarly the thermostat causes the heating system to be turned on again when the room temperature drops below 63°F (17°C).

The blood sugar is regulated in an analogous fashion. The system is illustrated by a large pot into which digested food particles flow. A blood sugar sensor acknowledges the rise in glucose concentration following food-intake rich in carbo-

function of
the pancreas

hydrates. It signals the pancreas to produce insulin and the pancreas then reacts by secreting insulin into the blood stream. As can be seen in the drawing, insulin now causes a "door" in the regulatory system to be opened, allowing the sugar to be directed out of the blood stream. Glucose can now flow into the liver, muscles or fatty tissues. The blood sugar drops to its normal level. At the same time the signal which the blood sugar sensor has been sending to the pancreas is interrupted. No further insulin is secreted and the "door" in the regulatory system is again closed. In this manner, the blood sugar concentration of a

11

healthy person is kept within the desired narrow limits.

Abnormal Sugar Metabolism

What are the consequences of the abnormal metabolism of a diabetic? The regulatory mechanism of his system is disrupted by the lack or insufficient production of insulin. When the diabetic consumes carbohydrates, the blood sugar concentration rises. Even though the blood sugar sensor registers this increase, the signal it sends to the pancreas does not cause a reaction, or one that is insufficient. As a result, the regulatory "door" is not opened or is only barely opened, completely or partially preventing the blood sugar from flowing into the blood stream.

the blood sugar rises

The blood sugar level continues to rise under these circumstances. After reaching a certain volume in the pot, which represents the circulatory system, the blood sugar must spill over. Blood sugar can now no longer serve the system as a source of energy.

The conditions in the diabetic's body are similar. When the blood sugar level rises too high, that is above 160 to 180 mg/l00ml, then the kidney begins losing part of the glucose with the urine. This critical borderline value is called the renal threshold. When the blood sugar level rises above this mark, sugar is found in the urine.

urinary sugar

The drawing also indicates the most important complaints and medical findings of the diabetic, which will be discussed in detail later. Two of these factors have been mentioned several times already: the elevated blood sugar level and the excretion of sugar in the urine.

The excess sugar can be found in the urine only if it is dissolved in plenty of water. Greater amounts of sugar can therefore be excreted only if the volume of urine is greater. The necessary water comes from the body and its cells. Since the water is almost forcefully taken from the body cells, the lack of water in the tissues leads to thirst and must be compensated by

thirst due to lack of water

fluid intake. Our model thus indicates two of the major symptoms of the untreated diabetic: frequent urination and thirst.

The drawing also allows us to explain the fatigue, decreased energy level and initial weight loss of the diabetic. Excess glucose flows through the blood stream into the kidney and out

12

with the urine. The glucose is therefore not available as a source of energy to the muscles. The muscles then suffer from a lack of energy, causing the diabetic to feel tired and faint.

Since the body must maintain its vital functions, it utilizes its energy reserves. The liver glycogen (a reserve consisting of glucose) is quickly depleted. Next, the reserves in the fatty tissue are used until little such tissue is left. This process causes the symptoms of weight loss and decreased energy level.

increased
acetone a
warning
signal

The fats in the fatty tissues cannot be burned up completely in the liver due to the lack of insulin. Intermediary products, the ketone bodies, are formed and build up in the body. (Three ketones are acetone, betahydroxybutyrate and acetoacetate.) They are excreted with urine in the form of acetone. A large amount of acetone in the urine is usually a sign of a serious disorder. The result of this situation may be hyperacidity of the blood and a life-threatening complication of diabetes, the diabetic coma.

Insulin deficiency is always decisive in diabetes mellitus: this hormone plays a major role in diabetes. But what causes this failure of the pancreas to produce insulin? In the following paragraphs we shall try to explain the natural history and the precipitating factors of diabetes. The term "natural history" refers to the development of the physical disorders which cause diabetes. Precipitating factors are external influences and conditions which bring about the acceleration of diabetes from an early to an advanced stage.

Natural History

diabetes,
a "family
disease"?

More than 95% of all cases of diabetes are caused by hereditary factors. Thus, diabetes is a genetically determined disorder. This observation sounds very definite, but it actually oversimplifies this condition, which is still not completely understood. It is not the disease, but rather the predisposition to develop diabetes which is inherited. Today, geneticists are certain (although some details remain to be explained) that the diabetic inherits the predisposition to develop diabetes. The fact that relatives of earlier generations did not suffer from diabetes is not sufficient counterevidence.

Other factors which lead to the development of diabetes

mellitus are found in less than 5% of all diabetics and are so obvious that they cannot be mistaken. Among these is the so-called "endocrine diabetes mellitus" resulting from a disease of the hormone glands, such as a tumor of the pituitary gland. (The pituitary gland is located at the base of the brain and one of its functions is to regulate other hormone glands.) Furthermore, if more than nine tenths of the insulin producing cells of the pancreas are destroyed in an accident or during severe illness, diabetes will result. This form of diabetes is pancreatic diabetes.

special forms of diabetes

Precipitating Factors

The genetic predisposition to develop diabetes does *not* in itself cause diabetes. Numerous external factors have a decisive influence in actually triggering the development and manifestation of the disease.

elevated risk with obesity

Obesity is the primary precipitating factor. The risk of developing diabetes in the presence of a genetic predisposition is multiplied by a factor of from 5 to 10 if weight is gained. In times of famine, the number of diabetics is much lower than in times of prosperity. About 90% of adults who have diabetes are overweight!

Precipitating factors of diabetes mellitus
- Overweight and overeating
- Pregnancy
- Infections
- Liver diseases
- Certain drugs

The development of diabetes in the presence of a genetic predisposition is hastened and advanced by the following factors:
- "Normal" changes in the interplay of hormone glands as for example in pregnancy.
- Unusual strain as in the case of severe infections which cause diabetes in about 10% of diabetics. All research done on infections indicates that they precipitate, but do not cause, diabetes.

- Chronic hepatitis, cirrhosis of the liver and other liver diseases often lead to diabetic disorders.
- The intake of certain kinds of drugs such as cortisone and its derivatives can trigger the development of diabetes. (*Cortisone* and its derivatives are chemical substances which correspond to the hormones produced by the adrenal cortex.) Cortisones may be found in drugs for rheumatism, asthma and hay fever.
- Diseases of the adrenal cortex which cause increased amounts of hormones to be produced. (The *adrenal cortex* is the outer part of the adrenal gland which produces hormones, as does the inner part or medulla.)
- The intake of medication against water-retention (called *diuretics*) and the birth control pill over a longer period of time. Most diabetics are aware that these drugs have a detrimental influence on the metabolism.

2. How to Diagnose Diabetes

Diabetes is a disease which is not always recognized immediately. Many diabetics become aware of their disease only gradually. These patients either have no complaints whatever or they may ignore disorders because they are not serious. Diabetes is often present for prolonged periods without being recognized as such. This is a potentially dangerous situation. Any diabetic, even if he has only slight complaints or none at all, must be treated. The grave complications of diabetes, the vascular diseases, can be prevented only if the metabolism is permanently normalized. Early recognition of diabetes is therefore one of the most important tasks of medicine. An estimated 4 million persons living in the United States are diabetic without knowing it, because the symptoms are not yet noticeable.

4 million Americans undiagnosed diabetics

15

Frequency of appearance for:

	juvenile-onset diabetes	adult-onset diabetes
Thirst	91%	67%
Loss of energy	80%	51%
Increased urination	75%	40%
Weight loss	72%	32%
Blurred vision	25%	28%
Itching	21%	22%

Chief Complaints and Results of Medical Tests.

The typical complaints of the untreated diabetic can hardly be confused with the symptoms of any other disease. The frequency of these symptoms varies greatly, as does their intensity and their development. The most frequent complaint is thirst. The more recently manifested diabetic patient complains slightly less frequently of a loss of energy and increased urination. Another frequent symptom is weight loss in the early stage. Numerous less common complaints include blurred vision and itching. It is therefore often the eye doctor or dermatologist who first makes the diagnosis of diabetes.

findings for diagnosis of diabetes

Even if the complaints noted are typical for a diabetic, the presumption or suspicion of diabetes must be followed by medical evidence. Obviously, an elevated blood sugar and the presence of sugar in the urine indicate diabetes. These symptoms must be treated, as must the frequent obesity and elevated levels of cholesterol and triglycerides.

The actual complications of long-term diabetes are changes in the eyes, disruptions in the kidney function, EKG abnormalities, circulatory and sensory disturbances (such as tingling) in the lower legs and feet. These symptoms must be expected in the first complete examination for diabetes, because the patient may have been suffering from this ailment for some time without his knowledge, thus allowing complications to develop.

What is examined	normal or desirable value
fasting blood sugar	up to 100 mg/100 ml
post-prandial blood sugar	up to 140 mg/100 ml
urinary sugar	not detectable
acetone in urine	not detectable
weight in kilograms	normal or ideal weight
cholesterol	below 200 mg/100 ml
triglyceride	below 150 mg/100 ml
systolic blood pressure	100 to 139 mm Hg
diastolic blood pressure	60 to 89 mm Hg

Examinations of the heart, kidneys, eyes, blood vessels and testing the function of the nervous system should be performed when the disease is first diagnosed and at regular intervals (for example, once a year) thereafter.

Warning Signs and Indicators

Latent diabetes causes *no* symptoms. Nevertheless, certain signs can indicate whether there is a genetic predisposition for potential development of diabetes. It takes a little detective work to acquire this information: facts must be gathered concerning illnesses of relatives and one's own personal disease history.

this also concerns your relatives

It is, of course, not always possible to determine if relatives were diabetic. Moreover, many people suffered from mild diabetes which was not detected in earlier times and ancestors with a strong genetic predisposition for diabetes may have died before developing symptoms. Nevertheless, the family history can provide important information. Seemingly unrelated facts noted in the family history, such as birth of an unusually large baby or complications in pregnancy for female relatives, as well as the occurrence of stroke, heart attack or high blood pressure may indicate a tendency of your family to develop diabetes. A family tendency toward other metabolic disorders which have a genetic origin, such as obesity or gout, must be noted because these problems often occur together with diabetes. Such family histories are significant, not only for you, but also for your relatives. They should also undergo medical examinations in order to allow the undiscovered diabetes to be recognized in an early stage and to prevent its further progression.

Checklist: indicators of diabetes

1. Is one of your blood relatives (parents, grandparents, brothers and sisters, children) a diabetic?
   Did he suffer from juvenile-onset or maturity-onset diabetes?

2. Did any of your relatives give birth to an unusually large child weighing more than 10 pounds at birth?

3. Do or did any of your blood relatives suffer from stroke heart attack or cardiac arrest,
   obesity,
   high blood pressure,
   gout,
   disorders of fat metabolism?

4. Did you ever experience "temporary" diabetes (for example, following an operation, during pregnancy or serious illness)? "Temporary" diabetes is latent diabetes which is manifest only under stress.
   Did you ever have urinary sugar during pregnancy, problems during pregnancy (children weighing more than 10 pounds, miscarriages)?
   Unusual results from a blood sugar test?

5. Do you suffer from
   obesity,
   thirst,
   increased urination,
   loss of energy,
   weight loss?
   Do you have itching in the genital region.
   blurred vision,
   gout,
   a problem in fat metabolism?

We mentioned important warning signs in the patient's history when we discussed the complications of diabetes. These symptoms — thirst, frequent urination, weight loss, and loss of energy — can develop so gradually that the patient may not notice changes. The patient often does not associate other bothersome complaints such as itching or small boils with diabetes.

18

From the Early Stages to the Actual Disease

The patient passes through different phases as the disease progresses from the genetic predisposition to the final illness.

Stages of diabetes mellitus
- Potential diabetes
- Latent diabetes
- Preclinical or asymptomatic diabetes
- Manifest diabetes

early stages of diabetes

Potential diabetes is the earliest stage which cannot yet be discovered with medical tests. Potential diabetes is presumed in a patient whose parents are both diabetic or in one who is the healthy identical twin of a diabetic. Moreover, women giving birth to children of more than 10 pounds are presumed to be diabetic.

In the stage of latent or asymptomatic diabetes, disorders of carbohydrate metabolism can be detected only by a special test, the so-called glucose tolerance test with a glucose load over 3 or even 5 hours. Preventive treatment should begin at this stage.

Recognition of the Early Stages

The early stages can be detected by tests, based on the fact that pancreatic function is limited even in this early stage. The pancreas is capable of producing the normal daily insulin requirement, but cannot meet additional demand. In the medical test, we artificially increase the demand by administering a large dose of glucose orally. The patient suspected of diabetes may not eat breakfast on the test day and must drink 100 grams of glucose dissolved in 400 milliliters of water or tea. If the highest blood sugar value exceeds 180 mg per 100 ml, and in particular if the blood sugar exceeds 140 mg per 100 ml after two hours following the initial dose, it is assumed that the patient is in an early stage of diabetes. This discovery is important because prevention must begin immediately. If the patient is overweight, he must lose weight, hopefully attaining normal weight. Normal weight patients must take care not to gain weight.

glucose tolerance test

It is not necessary to perform a glucose tolerance test in the case of manifest diabetes with elevated blood sugar *and* sugar present in the urine.

3. Types of Diabetes

Different kinds of diabetes are distinguished by degree of insulin production, age of the patient when disease is discovered, and by the required method of treatment.

Types of diabetes	Discovery of the disease
Childhood diabetes	up to age 14
Juvenile-onset diabetes	ages 15 to 24
Maturity-onset diabetes	ages 25 to 65
Diabetes in old age	after age 65

Juvenile-Onset Diabetes

absolute
insulin
deficiency

In the case of absolute insulin deficiency, the patient must undergo injections of this substance for the rest of his life. We will call this insulin-deficiency, juvenile-onset diabetes and include all forms of diabetes in adolescents in this group. This patient tends to be slender when the disease develops. After a longer period of time, one in two adolescents becomes overweight.

No insulin production = juvenile-onset diabetes (absolute insulin deficiency) = permanent insulin treatment (and diet) necessary.

Maturity-Onset Diabetes

In contrast to the patient with juvenile-onset diabetes, the patient with maturity-onset diabetes has insufficient reserves of insulin. More than 90% of all diabetics are included in this type. They are usually obese. These patients can almost always be treated with a combination of diet and oral hypoglycemic agents.

Insufficient production of insulin = maturity-onset diabetes (relative insulin deficiency) = diet (and possibly oral hypoglycemic agents) usually necessary.

After a longer period of illness, the relative insulin deficiency of the patient can become so severe that insulin administration is necessary.

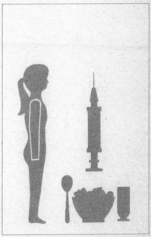

"Which Type of Diabetes Do I Have?"

The patient should determine which type of diabetes he has, and then read about the methods of treatment required. The choice of the method of treatment is determined not only by the type of insulin deficiency — absolute or relative — but also by weight and age of patient.

An obese adult diabetic, for example, must be treated differently than a slender diabetic child. The methods of treatment lead to different prognoses.

The types of diabetes can be differentiated by the incidence rate; for example, obese adult diabetics are very frequent, while obese diabetic children are rare. Naturally, different treatment methods must be used in each classification.

Before we begin to discuss practical suggestions for diabetes treatment, the patient should know which type of diabetes he has and which treatment methods must be emphasized.

The strict differentiation between 10 different types of diabetes allows the patient to find the appropriate measures of treatment.

I am:
- **a diabetic child**
- without endogenic insulin
- normal-weight
- treated with insulin and diet

The diabetic child must inject insulin daily because of the absolute lack of endogenic insulin. A balance must be found between nutrition, physical activity and insulin administration. Treatment should be individualized on the basis of frequent and regular tests of the metabolism to suit individual needs.

What I have to know:
- good diabetes control (p. 32)
- diabetes diet (p. 36)
- insulin treatment (p. 70)
- physical activity (p. 77)
- self-testing of metabolism (p. 87)
- the "diabetic child" (p. 107)
- choice of career (p. 101)

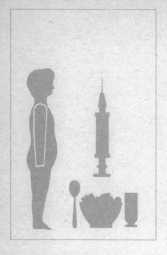 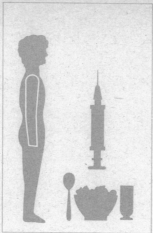 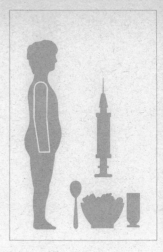

I am:
- **a diabetic child**
- without endogenic insulin
- overweight
- treated with insulin and diet
- I should lose weight

The diabetic child must inject insulin daily because of the absolute insulin deficiency. The correct balance must be found between nutrition, physical activity and insulin administration, and exact quantities of each can be determined by the results of the regular self-testing. Normal weight should be attained.

What I have to know:
- good diabetes control (p. 32)
- diabetes diet (p. 36)
- weight reduction (p. 75)
- administration of insulin (p. 70)
- physical activity (p. 77)
- self-testing of blood and urinary sugar (p. 87)
- "the diabetic child" (p. 107)
- choice of career (p. 101)

I am:
- **a patient with juvenile-onset diabetes**
- without endogenic insulin
- normal weight
- treated with insulin and diet

The adolescent diabetic must also inject insulin daily due to the absolute insulin deficiency. A balance must be found between nutrition, physical activity and administration of insulin. All measures of treatment can be individualized according to the results of regular self-testing.

What I have to know:
- good diabetes control (p. 32)
- diabetes diet (p. 36)
- administration of insulin (p. 70)
- physical activity (p. 77)
- self-testing of blood and urinary sugar (p. 87)
- choice of career (p. 101)
- relationships, sexuality, family planning (p. 97)
- driver's license (p. 103)

I am:
- **a patient with juvenile-onset diabetes**
- without endogenic insulin
- overweight
- treated with insulin and diet
- I want to lose weight

The adolescent diabetic must inject insulin daily due to the absolute insulin deficiency. A balance must be found between nutrition, physical activity and administration of insulin. Treatment may be individualized according to the results of regular self-testing. Maintaining normal weight is important for bringing the blood and urinary sugar under control.

What I need to know:
- good diabetes control (p. 32)
- diabetes diet (p. 36)
- administration of insulin (p. 70)
- weight reduction (p. 75)
- physical activity (p. 77)
- self-testing of blood and urinary sugar (p. 87)
- choice of career (p. 101)
- relationships, sexuality, family planning (p. 97)
- driver's license (p. 103)

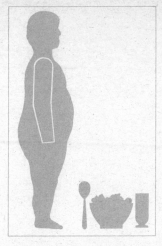 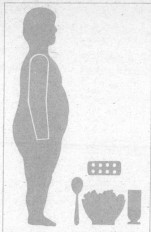 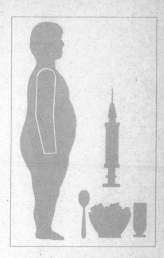

I am:
- **a patient with maturity-onset diabetes**
- with endogenic insulin
- overweight
- treated with diet
- I want to lose weight

It is often possible to treat obese adult diabetics with diet alone. The diet must take the relative deficiency of endogenic insulin into account, making numerous small meals and weight reduction necessary. The obese diabetic should lose weight even if the blood sugar and urinary sugar tests show normal results. Since the overweight condition strains the pancreas, drug therapy with oral hypoglycemic agents or insulin becomes necessary after a certain period of time.

What I have to know:
- good diabetes control (p. 32)
- diabetes diet (p. 36)
- weight reduction (p. 75)
- physical activity (p. 77)

I am:
- **a patient with maturity-onset diabetes**
- with endogenic insulin
- overweight
- treated with diet and oral hypoglycemic agents
- I want to lose weight

Most diabetics fall into this category. Although the obese adult diabetic may have endogenic insulin, this insulin is not sufficient to cover the demands made by obesity. The obese adult diabetic must lose weight, because then his own insulin reserves will be sufficient to meet the normal weight requirements. Drug therapy is no longer necessary.

What I must know:
- good diabetes control (p. 32)
- diabetes diet (p. 36)
- weight reduction (p. 75)
- treatment with oral hypoglycemic agents (p. 66)
- physical activity (p. 77)

I am:
- **a patient with maturity-onset diabetes**
- with endogenic insulin
- overweight
- treated with diet and insulin
- I want to lose weight
- perhaps I will not need additional insulin then

This group of obese adult diabetics must inject insulin to ensure good metabolic functioning despite the fact that they still produce endogenic insulin. These endogenic reserves of insulin are not sufficient to meet the demands made by obesity on the metabolism. When these diabetics lose weight, they usually need no further insulin injections because their own reserves are sufficient and can be mobilized by means of oral hypoglycemic agents.

What I must know:
- good diabetes control (p. 32)
- diabetes diet (p. 36)
- weight reduction (p. 75)
- administration of insulin (p. 70)
- self-testing of urinary and blood sugar (p. 87)
- physical activity (p. 77)
- (perhaps later) treatment with oral hypoglycemic agents (p. 66)

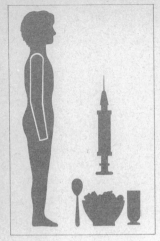 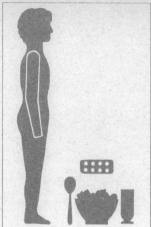 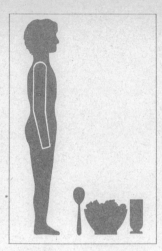

I am:
- **a patient with maturity-onset diabetes**
- with insufficient endogenic insulin
- normal weight
- treated with diet and insulin

Some older normal-weight diabetics produce less endogenic insulin as the years go by, and therefore must be treated with daily insulin injections. Diet and physical activity must be adapted to these injections and can be individualized according to the results of the self-testing.

What I need to know:
- good diabetes control (p. 32)
- diabetes diet (p. 36)
- administration of insulin (p. 70)
- physical activity (p. 77)
- self-testing of urinary and blood sugar (p. 87)

I am:
- **a patient with maturity-onset diabetes**
- with endogenic insulin
- normal weight
- treated with diet and oral hypoglycemic agents

These normal weight adult diabetics who are treated with oral hypoglycemic agents and diet should be careful not to gain weight. Only then can they maintain the normalization of their diabetes. Sometimes more serious disorders of the metabolism appear as indicated by elevated blood sugar levels despite a correct diet and treatment with oral hypoglycemic agents; this would make insulin administration necessary.

What I must know:
- good diabetes control (p. 32)
- diabetes diet (p. 36)
- physical activity (p. 77)
- treatment with oral hypoglycemic agents (p. 66)

I am:
- **a patient with maturity-onset diabetes**
- with endogenic insulin
- normal weight
- treated with diet

This is an "ideal case" of diabetes because the normal weight adult diabetic can be treated with diet alone. Many obese adult diabetics who must be treated with oral hypoglycemic agents can be placed in this category once they lose weight. Diabetics in this category should maintain their normal weight in order to avoid a deterioration of their metabolism which would make drug therapy necessary.

What I must know:
- good diabetes control (p. 32)
- diabetes diet (p. 36)

4. Acute Effects and Damaging Sequelae

The Diabetic Coma

The diabetic coma determined the fate of the diabetic up until 60 years ago, when insulin was discovered. A coma is defined as deep prolonged unconsciousness. Doctors were helpless as they watched the diabetic's condition continue to deteriorate, until the patient's death.

It was clear the first time that diabetes was treated with insulin that this discovery was a true blessing. The 14 year old Leonard Thompson was lying in a hospital in Toronto on January 11, 1922. He had been diabetic for almost two years and was now close to death, completely emaciated, dehydrated, and unconscious. He felt better after only one injection of insulin and recuperated quickly within the next few days, after which he was able to lead a normal life with the help of insulin.

The type of diabetic coma experienced by this boy during that period prior to 1922 was almost always fatal. The diabetic coma is still fatal today if the patient is left untreated. However, the coma can be prevented if an attempt is made to bring the blood sugar level under control.

life-saving insulin

The Uncontrolled Metabolic Disorder

The diabetic must know when his life is endangered because the threat of coma exists. The diabetic should become familiar with the signs indicating that the metabolic disorder is so severe that over a prolonged length of time a coma may become inevitable. The four warning signs include:

- thirst
- increased urination
- fatigue and loss of energy
- weight loss

25

We mentioned these chief complaints in the discussion of symptoms. They are always signs of a serious metabolic disorder even if the diabetes is under treatment.

the Greeks knew of diabetes

Greek physicians diagnosed and described this condition as far back as the period of classical antiquity: "melting down of flesh and limbs to urine ... It is not posssible to stop the flood and it is as if a water pipe has broken open ... The thirst cannot be quenched". (This is a quotation from Aretaeus, who was probably the first to use the term diabetes.) A patient who notices any of these warning signs must consult a physician immediately.

Symptoms of the Coma

The metabolic disorder can progress from well-being into a diabetic coma very quickly. The coma is caused by an absolute insulin deficiency at that particular moment. Neither fat nor sugar metabolism is under control.

Not only is the body forcefully dehydrated, but it is also flooded with ketone bodies, which are the acidic intermediary products of fat metabolism. The consequences, dehydration and hyperacidity of the blood and tissues, lead to loss of consciousness.

symptoms of a developing coma

How can the development of this acute danger be detected? These warning signs of metabolic disorder and the following symptoms indicate the onset of a diabetic coma:

- nausea
- vomiting
- abdominal pain
- the smell of acetone in exhaled air

The smell of exhaled acetone is similar to that of rotten apples or nail polish. The body is trying to expel part of the acid, or ketone bodies, by exhalation and urination.

The diabetic coma can be prevented. To avoid a coma, the diabetic must not only know the symptoms of a severe metabolic disorder but must also be on guard for the factors which most commonly precipitate coma:

factors which trigger a coma

- inflammation and infectious diseases
- heart attack

26

- stroke
- other problems from vascular diseases
- improper diet
- insufficient administration of insulin
- undiscovered or untreated diabetes

Anyone who develops these warning signs must be admitted to a hospital immediately. However, diabetics today should never develop coma. This dangerous condition can only be prevented by bringing the blood sugar levels under control

Decreased Blood Sugar Level — Hypoglycemia — Shock

the opposite type of metabolic disorder

The opposite of an elevated blood sugar level lapsing into coma is the decreased blood sugar level which leads to hypoglycemia.

A sharp decrease in the blood sugar level of an insulin-dependent diabetic is called shock. This state is caused by unbalanced treatment when the blood-sugar lowering effect of insulin is too strong. The blood sugar level drops abruptly causing hypoglycemia because the carbohydrate intake was insufficient compared to the amount of insulin. The specific complaints will be discussed in greater detail later, because hypoglycemia is a side effect of diabetes treatment and can be understood only with reference to the treatment as a whole.

Harmful Consequences of Diabetes

The diabetic does not die from his diabetes, but from the harmful consequences of the disease. The most frequent causes of death are vascular diseases such as heart attack or stroke. The incidence of these diseases increases when diabetes is poorly treated, thus decreasing the patient's life expectancy.

dying from the conse-quences

The incidence of vascular damage and its consequences, particularly heart attack and stroke, are especially frequent in diabetics.

Undoubtedly, our modern life-style plays an important role. "We were healthier when things were not so easy for us." Obviously, the standard of living is higher and with it, physical

27

activity has drastically decreased over the past century and food is more plentiful.

what are
risk-factors?

This brings us to the topic of risk factors which affect diabetic patients. What is a risk factor? Since many renowned physicians have already answered this question, we quote one of them:

"If you drive under the influence of alcohol, then you increase the risk of a traffic accident. The elevated alcohol content of your blood becomes a risk factor for you. Or if your child suffers from chronic tonsillitis, then this condition may cause rheumatic carditis and arthritis or renal disease: the tonsillitis is a risk factor." (Quote from Dr. Wolff, *Speaking of High Blood Pressure*.)

In medical usage, a disorder leading to certain diseases is called a risk factor. These include not only medical conditions, but also environmental factors. The term risk factor is used in epidemiology, the study of the frequency of certain diseases in a population. This research has found a relationship between certain risk factors and the development of cardio-vascular disease. Epidemiological studies have shown that persons who suffered from heart attack or stroke had certain risk factors which persons whose heart and blood vessel systems were healthy did not have.

Common Blood Vessel Diseases

Diabetes is a risk factor in the development of vascular damage, which may lead to serious diseases. Diabetic patients tend to suffer more frequently than healthy persons from blood vessel diseases in various organs. More specifically, the arterial walls undergo certain changes if the blood and urinary sugar are not brought under control. The arteries become narrowed, allowing less blood to flow through them. Tissues and organs which have been well-supplied with the vital oxygen carrying blood now

late
sequelae:
arterio-
sclerosis

suffer from inadequate blood and oxygen supply. These changes take place in the small vessels, particularly in the kidneys and eyes. A higher incidence of hardening of the arteries, called arteriosclerosis, one of the most frequent causes of death in the population as a whole, is found in diabetics at an earlier age. (*Arteriosclerosis* is the medical term for development of narrowing of the arteries.) In serious cases, such vascular damage leads to severe disease such as blindness, chronic

28

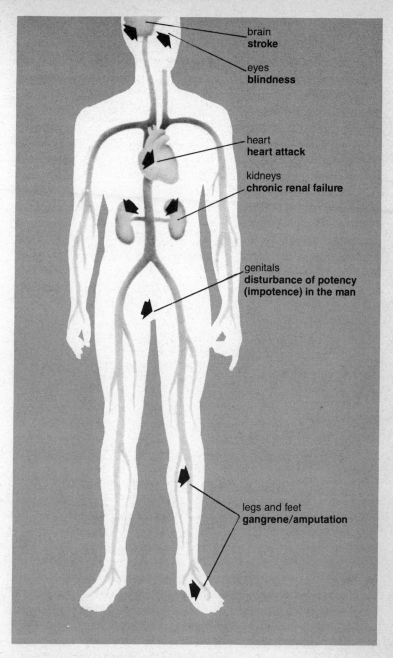

brain
stroke

eyes
blindness

heart
heart attack

kidneys
chronic renal failure

genitals
**disturbance of potency
(impotence) in the man**

legs and feet
gangrene/amputation

The harmful consequences of diabetes. Diabetics are more likely to develop circulatory disorders than are healthy persons. In severe cases, the vascular damage is fatal. The extent of harmful consequences can be limited by correct treatment.

kidney failure, heart attack, stroke, and gangrene of the feet (see illustration). (*Gangrene* is literally death and decay of tissue in a toe or limb due to failure of blood and oxygen supply.)

Information on risk factors for diabetes can help the diabetic improve his treatment. The diabetic can decrease his risk factors in a decisive way if he can bring his blood sugar under control, avoid sugar in the urine and maintain this normalized state. Such control plays an essential role in decreasing risk of vascular disease.

Diabetics are threatened not only by the "classical" risk factors, the vascular diseases, but also by other related diseases which may appear in combination. These related diseases resemble vascular damage, as they, too, are influenced by the metabolic disorder: they are less frequent in diabetics whose blood and urinary sugar is brought under control. Among these related problems are skin infections such as small boils and athlete's foot; bothersome itching occurring especially in the vagina for women; kidney disease and infections of the urethra and the bladder; diseases of the gall bladder and liver, such as gall stones or fatty liver degeneration.

Diabetics often develop several of these complaints resulting from neuropathies simultaneously. Sensory disturbances in arms and legs, such as inability to feel pain, also belong to this category.

In the course of his disease, one in two diabetics may experience a disturbance of sexual function. Often, embarrassment wrongly leads the patient to avoid discussing this topic with the physician. As a result, the diabetic is plagued by psychological and marital problems, although the complaints can usually be treated. A basic prerequisite for improvement is bringing the blood sugar under excellent control.

talk with your physician

Additional Risk Factors for Vascular Damage

Diabetes is only one of many risk factors for coronary and vascular disease. Further risk factors include:
- elevated blood cholesterol (hypercholesterolemia)
- cigarette smoking
- high blood pressure (hypertension)
- elevated uric acid (hyperuricemia)
- gout
- (indirectly) obesity

The significance of these risk factors is clear: they precipitate and reinforce the development of arteriosclerosis by changing the walls of the arterial blood vessels. The vessels become so rigid and narrow that the blood supply to organs is impaired or interrupted. The result, as previously indicated, may be heart attack, stroke, or large blood vessel disease in the legs.

success with
treatment
possible

All risk factors must be treated and prevented if possible. Treatment of risk factors is not just the doctor's order, but a concrete chance the patient has to improve his condition. Do not be frightened by this discussion of harmful consequences of diabetes. These descriptions are intended to make you more aware of potential problems with your health. Risk factors such as high blood pressure, gout, and disturbances of fat metabolism can be successfully treated in the diabetic. Some of them can be removed permanently, thus eliminating the risk after a certain period of time — you should be able to do so in the cases of cigarette smoking and obesity.

5. Successful Treatment of Diabetes

Physician-Patient Cooperation

Cooperation with the physician makes it possible to realize the goal of bringing the urinary and blood sugar levels under control and eliminating sugar from the urine. The physician and patient share the task of treatment.

treatment of
diabetes in-
volves long-
term therapy

In a successful program for diabetes treatment, the physician's function is to prescribe an individual treatment plan for the patient. The doctor may find it necessary to modify this plan in

31

the course of regular check-ups.

It is the patient's responsibility to adhere to and comply with the medical treatment plan each day. The success of long-term therapy depends upon the patient's willingness to understand and to relate the results of his self-testing to the physician, as well as on his conscientious attempt to work together with the physician.

The physician can provide correct advice only if the patient informs him of all results of his self-testing in the time period between medical consultations. These considerations are basic to the following chapters. No differentiation is made between daily measures undertaken for treatment:

- the physician determines the treatment method and
- the diabetic treats himself.

Good Diabetes Control Is Decisive

Every diabetic must make a daily attempt to bring his blood sugar under control. It is impossible otherwise to prevent such dangerous complications as hypoglycemia and coma. Bringing the blood sugar under control and eliminating sugar from the urine is the only way these harmful consequences can be prevented or diminished to allow the patient to lead a normal life.

Good diabetes control leads to the following results:

any diabetic can do it

- physical and emotional well-being;
- capacity to lead a normal active life;
- participation in family, professional and social life;
- higher life expectancy

What is entailed in bringing the blood sugar level under control? Ideally, the metabolic disorder is brought under control so effectively that the diabetic can no longer be distinguished from a healthy person. You should always try to meet this goal. But do not do so merely to please the physician for the next medical consultation. Many diabetics deceive themselves by making special attempts in the few days before the medical examination only to neglect the treatment after the examination because the medical findings were "good". This means that urine and blood sugar levels had been brought under control for only two or three days.

Effective control of the blood sugar level requires a carefully and permanently balanced system. A daily attempt must be made to meet normal values for blood sugar and avoidance of sugar in the urine.

leading a better life with good diabetes control

This result calls for willpower and determination on the patient's part. The patient will be encouraged by the good results he can expect to achieve. The reward for complete control of the blood sugar level is prevention of the most dangerous complication, diabetic coma. The diabetic will then be able to avoid the complaints associated with elevated blood sugar values, such as thirst, increased urination, itching, weakness, tingling or blurred vision. These usually disappear completely upon gaining control of the blood sugar level.

save on medication

Obese diabetics can easily bring the blood sugar levels under control by losing weight. Weight reduction may enable the diabetic to become less dependent on oral hypoglycemic tablets. Often obese diabetics who must inject insulin discover that they can manage without these injections and can use a combination of diet and oral agents instead. Some diabetics no longer require any oral hypoglycemic agents when they lose weight.

Good diabetes control, combined with weight reduction, has a decisive influence on the obese diabetic. About 90% of the 9 million diabetics living in the U.S. are obese. If the weight of all these patients were reduced, then millions of dollars spent on medications could be saved.

The savings possible should be an incentive toward achievement of at least some weight loss. Often a 20 pound weight reduction will allow you to avoid increasing doses of medication or changing from treatment with oral hypoglycemic agents to treatment with insulin.

the most important goal of treatment

The most important goal of diabetic treatment is to avoid or delay the harmful consequences to the vascular system. This reason is probably not a sufficient motivation for all diabetics because the threat of a future danger is usually not enough to induce preventive measures now.

Nonetheless, the most important goal and the essence of diabetic treatment is bringing the blood sugar level under control. A comparison between normalized and abnormal metabolism will

33

show that vascular damage and its consequences can be prevented to a large degree.

Goals of good diabetes control

benefits

Effective treatment of diabetes should:
• Prevent exacerbation of the disease;
• Guarantee that acute dangers do not arise;
• Help avoid or delay vascular damage.

By means of good treatment the diabetic attains:
• Physical and emotional well-being;
• Normal capacity to lead an active life;
• Unimpaired participation in family, professional and social life;
• A normal life-expectancy.

Guidelines for Diabetes Control

self-testing

What practical daily measures should the diabetic take to bring his blood sugar under control? How is a balanced metabolism distinguished from an abnormal one? Diabetes specialists have agreed to certain values as criteria for normalization (see table). These guidelines allow the patient to check for himself, either after a medical exam or during self-testing at home, whether or not the goals have been met. Please note that a single value (for example, blood sugar) is not sufficient by itself to allow reliable judgment. All medical examinations must include testing of blood and urinary sugar (possibly for acetone) and body weight; all self-examinations must include testing of urinary sugar (possibly for acetone) and body weight. The physician should examine the blood lipids, cholesterol and triglycerides, and if necessary the uric acid and blood pressure.

Guidelines for good diabetes control

For patients who are treated either with insulin or else with a combination of insulin and oral hypoglycemic agents.

Fasting glucose:

normal	up to 120 mg/100 ml
clearly abnormal	above 150 mg/100 ml

Postprandial glucose tolerance:

normal	up to 160 mg/100 ml
clearly abnormal	above 200 mg/100 ml

Urinary sugar excretion per 24 hours:

normal	none
clearly abnormal	above 10 grams

Acetone in urine:

normal	none
abnormal	negative/positive

Cholesterol:

normal	up to 220 mg/100 ml
abnormal	over 250 mg/100 ml

Triglycerides:

normal	up to 150 mg/100 ml
abnormal	above 200 mg/100 ml

For patients who are treated with a combination of diet and insulin.

Fasting glucose:

normal	up to 140 mg/100 ml
clearly abnormal	above 170 mg/100 ml

Postprandial glucose tolerance:

normal	up to 180 mg/100 ml
clearly abnormal	above 230 mg/100 ml

Excretion of urinary sugar in 24 hours:

normal	up to 15 grams
clearly abnormal	above 25 grams

Acetone in urine:

normal	none
abnormal	negative/postive

Cholesterol:

normal	up to 220 mg/100 ml
abnormal	above 250 mg/100 ml

Triglycerides:

normal	up to 150 mg/100 ml
abnormal	above 200 mg/100 ml

Normal weight is absolutely essential for good diabetes control even if laboratory results are normal!

6. The Diabetes Diet: Adapted to Individual Needs

Looking back on the history of diabetes for thousands of years, we can see that today's patient is very fortunate. Few methods were available for treatment and most of them were of little use until insulin was discovered. Formerly the only methods of treatment available were based on certain restrictive diets. When the miraculous effects of insulin were first observed, it was thought that diet would no longer be an indispensable part of treatment because the insulin deficiency could now be regulated.

no success without diet

Physicians soon realized that insulin alone was not sufficient to normalize the metabolic disorder if a balanced diet was not included. Soon after the discovery of insulin, the famous American diabetes specialist, Professor E. P. Joslin was quick to point out that the living habits and life-style of the diabetic patient had to be changed to suit his metabolic needs. According to Joslin, whose opinion is still highly respected today, the three major elements of therapy must be diet, insulin and physical activity.

The Diet Is Basic

"Diet is basic to the treatment of diabetes" — "The proper nutrition of the diabetic is essential" — "If all of us were to eat the way diabetics should eat, the general health of the entire population would be better." Such remarks are made frequently. Whether the term "diet" or the words "proper nutrition" are used, is irrelevant because both mean the same thing. The diabetes diet is not a list of prohibited foods but rather a healthy, diversified and tasteful nutrition.

"Healthy nutrition" is a challenge to the average person to change his usual diet in favor of a healthier life-style.

practice these diet rules

The diabetic must meet the same challenge: he cannot simply eat whatever he would like whenever he would like in the quantity he desires. The diabetes diet imposes certain restrictions to which the diabetic must become accustomed. Words such as "should", "must", and "should not" are therefore often used in description of this diet.

Like other diabetics, you can also learn to apply and adhere to the diabetes diet. You will soon recognize the benefits.

Basics about the Nutritional Value of Various Foods

Before we can elaborate the principle of the diabetes diet, we must discuss the basic elements of nutrition. We have already discussed the basic components of food, the carbohydrates, fats (lipids) and proteins. These serve as building blocks for the body's own substances and are also a source of energy for the function of the body.

The important carbohydrates which we consume for energy are foods such as bread, flour, flour products, potatoes, rice, fruits and vegetables. These foods contain different types of sugar, glucose and fructose, which are absorbed at various rates by the body. The slower the carbohydrates are absorbed into the blood stream, the better they are for the diabetic. Glucose itself is a simple or pure carbohydrate. It passes into the blood stream quickly through the wall of the intestine and rapidly elevates the blood sugar level. For this reason, glucose and sugar are not suitable for the diabetic.

how the body absorbs carbohydrates

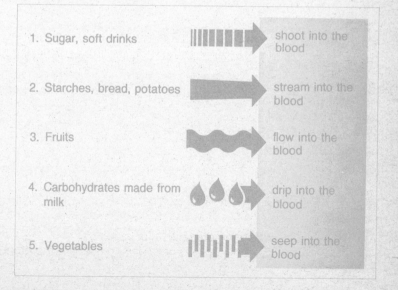

1. Sugar, soft drinks — shoot into the blood

2. Starches, bread, potatoes — stream into the blood

3. Fruits — flow into the blood

4. Carbohydrates made from milk — drip into the blood

5. Vegetables — seep into the blood

The fats we consume also serve primarily as an energy source and fats often contain vitamins. They appear in foods derived from both animals and vegetables. While some fats are visible, others are hidden. Examples of visible fats are butter, margarine, lard, oil and bacon. Hidden fats are found in meat, sausage, eggs, milk and milk products, fish and in nuts. Not all fats are the same. Foods which contain a higher level of polyunsaturated fats normalize the fat metabolism and lower an already elevated cholesterol level in the blood. Preference should be given to these fats which are found in certain margarines, safflower oil, soybean oil, corn oil or sunflower oil.

visible and hidden fats

Another fat-like substance, cholesterol, is found in cell walls and serves as a building-block for certain hormones. Since a high level of cholesterol in the blood promotes arteriosclerosis, the intake of this substance should be restricted. High amounts of cholesterol are contained in eggs, butter, lard, liver, kidney and brain, that is, in all meats from inner organs.

The building-blocks for substances which the body produces itself are contained in proteins found in animal and vegetable foods. Half of the daily protein requirement should consist of animal protein such as meat, fish, eggs, milk, and milk products. Vegetable protein is found in products from corn and grain, potatoes and other vegetables.

daily protein requirement

A healthy diet must include sufficient vegetables and minerals, neither of which is a source of energy. Important sources of vitamins are whole wheat bread, brown rice, milk, meat, fish, fruits, vegetables and potatoes. Minerals, vital substances which help to build the skeleton (bones and teeth) in children, are needed for cell structures and serve as building-blocks for enzymes and hormones. Most foods rich in vitamins also contain minerals.

Besides such digestible and vital elements, food also contains some elements which are not digestible, bulk materials. They pass through the intestines without being used and stimulate normal functioning of the intestines. Fruits, vegetables, whole wheat bread, wheat germ and bran contain useful bulk materials.

The Physician Establishes the Diet

All diet plans for diabetics should be based on insight gained from the study of nutrition and the metabolic disturbances of the

	Small Frame	Medium Frame	Large Frame
Weight in pounds in indoor clothing, with shoes.			
Men (over age 25)			
5'2"	112-120	118-129	126-141
5'4"	118-126	124-136	132-148
5'6"	124-133	130-143	138-156
5'8"	132-141	138-152	147-166
5'10"	140-150	146-160	155-174
6'0"	148-158	154-170	164-184
6'2"	156-167	162-180	173-194
6'4"	164-175	172-190	182-204
Women (Over age 25)			
4'10"	92-98	96-107	104-119
5'0"	96-104	101-113	109-125
5'2"	102-110	107-119	115-131
5'4"	108-116	113-126	121-138
5'6"	114-123	120-135	129-146
5'8"	122-131	128-143	137-154
5'10"	130-140	136-151	145-163

diabetic patient. There is no uniform diet which suits all such persons. Instead, the nutrition plan must be adapted to fit each individual's needs. In setting up such a plan, the doctor considers several different criteria which may vary from one patient to the next: age, sex, size, weight, and physical activity.

In order to determine the total calories which each diabetic may consume, one must know what the normal weight of the diabetic should be. The normal weight is associated with the longest life expectancy. Values used today are based upon studies made by American insurance companies (see chart above. The lower values would be *ideal* weights). A rule of thumb to find the normal weight in kilograms is to subtract 100 from the height expressed in centimeters. For example, a person 178 centimeters in height should weigh about 78 kilograms. The *ideal* weight is calculated by subtracting an additional 10% for men and 15% for women from this result. Thus, a man who is 178 cm. tall should ideally weigh about 70 kg. (1 kg. = 2.2 pounds.)

The total amount of food intake allowed per day is calculated

what is your
ideal weight?

39

Energy requirement of various activities

Light physical activity:	32 calories per 2 pounds (1 kg.) of weight
Average physical activity:	37 calories per 2 pounds (1 kg.) of weight
Heavy physical activity:	40-50 calories per 2 pounds (1 kg.) of weight

according to the ideal weight, or to be generous, according to the normal weight and the type of physical activity of the diabetic. Most persons, 75% of the population, perform only light physical work.

It has been generally agreed that intake of energy should be distributed among the basic nutrients as follows: 20% from protein, 35% from fat, and 45% from carbohydrates. Different foods can then be chosen within these three groups.

The daily allowance of food should be taken in several small meals per day. Since the pancreas produces only a small amount

blood sugar curve with six meals

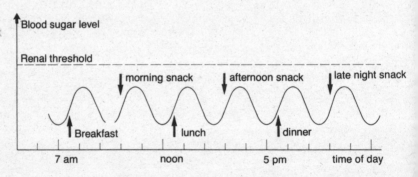

blood sugar curve with three meals

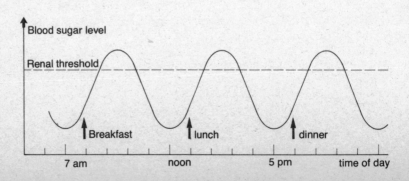

or perhaps no insulin at all, it can help in digestion of small meals only. Large meals make such a great demand on the metabolism of the diabetic that the blood sugar level is greatly elevated (see following chart). The analogy with a bridge which can carry only a 5 ton load will illustrate this situation. If six separate 5 ton trucks cross the bridge one after the other, then neither the bridge nor trucks are affected. But if one 30 ton truck or all 6 of the 5 ton trucks cross at the same time, then the bridge may collapse.

The physician will suggest six to seven small meals when he develops the diet plan. He will establish a balance between the distribution of food intake, the daily routine and amount of physical exertion, as well as the medical treatment. The snacks, midmorning, midafternoon or late night snack, may consist of fruit, bread or yogurt. These snacks can easily be consumed either at home or at the place of work.

The physician's calculations and considerations serve as the background for the diet plan which the diabetic patient must follow. This diet plan is no more than a frame of reference, as the following examples will show. The diabetic certainly is not forced to eat the same items each day: rather, he may exchange one food for another using the lists of substitute foods in order to bring more variety to the meals.

The Most Important Dietary Rules for the Diabetic

Although the physician establishes the diet plan for you, he cannot help you in actually executing the plan. Therefore you should always keep the following rules in mind:

Diet rules
1. Eat no more than necessary to maintain your ideal weight.
2. Distribute the daily food allowance among 6 or 7 meals.
3. Do not consume sugar or foods and drinks containing sugar or sweetened with sugar.
4. Limit the amount of fats in food.
5. Use the diet plan and scales for the precise calculation of food quantities.

Although these diet rules are applicable to all categories of diabetics, their significance varies from one diabetic to the next.

No insulin production = adolescent diabetes = constant insulin treatment = frequent small meals.

Insufficient production of insulin = adult diabetes = relieving the pancreas = weight reduction.

The distribution of carbohydrate intake over several meals per day (diet rule #2) is certainly the most important rule for the insulin dependent diabetic. But even if you do not need insulin, you should always find a way to limit yourself to several small meals per day.

If a diabetic consumes large amounts of carbohydrates as healthy people usually do with each meal of the day, then his blood sugar level will increase sharply since the metabolism is not normal. However, if he consumes small amounts more frequently, then the blood sugar level will increase within the normal limits.

better dia-
betes control
through
weight
reduction

The need to reduce weight (rules #1 and #4) is important, obviously, for the obese adult diabetic. But even a slender insulin dependent diabetic should be weight-conscious because any weight gain will immediately be translated into an unbalanced metabolism.

All diabetics should choose only those carbohydrates which are best for them (rule #3). Preferable foods are those containing carbohydrates which are absorbed slowly into the blood stream. The diabetic should avoid pure sugar which will lead to an immediate increase in the blood sugar level.

What the Diabetic Should and Should Not Eat

The first of the following two tables lists typical American foods which the diabetic must avoid. Since fast food chains and processed food plants are not yet required by the Food and Drug administration to reveal the exact ingredients, the nutritional value and calorie count of these foods can only be estimated. However, one can safely estimate that the amount of hidden fat in

Table 1

Examples of foods the diabetic must avoid

The diabetic should avoid typical examples of American food listed below because:
1. the caloric content is unknown and
2. they contain hidden amounts of animal fats, carbohydrates and salt.

Processed food
TV dinners
packaged foods in vending machines
foods from fast food chains
Ham and sausage biscuits
Hotdogs
Pizza
Cheeseburgers
Potato chips, fritos, etc.
French fries, hush puppies, etc.
Doughnuts
Milkshakes
Fried seafood
Salad dressing not low in calories

Other foods likely to cause problems:
Peanut butter and jelly sandwiches
Ice cream
Mayonnaise
Cake and cookies
Canned fruit in heavy syrup

Table 2

Diabetes diet
Limited to 1000 calories per day for the 90% of all diabetics who are obese.
Consult substitution lists at end of book for exchanging foods.

Breakfast
one fruit substitution
one bread substitution
one meat substitution
½ cup skim milk or equivalent from milk substitution
one fat substitution

Lunch
one meat substitution
two vegetable substitutions
one bread substitution
vegetables as desired from section 1 vegetables substitution list
one fruit substitution
½ cup skim milk or equivalent from milk substitution

Dinner
three meat substitutions
one bread substitution
one vegetable substitution
vegetables as desired from section 1 vegetable substitution list
½ fruit substitution
one fat substitution

Late night snack
one cup skim milk or
equivalent from milk substitution
OR
one fruit substitution and ½ bread substitution

Table 3

Example of 1000 calorie menu plan outlined in Table 2.

Food	Portion	Cal.
Breakfast (265 calories)		
coffee (without sugar)	as desired	0
skim milk	½ cup	40
orange juice	½ cup	40
toast	1 slice	70
egg	1	70
margarine	1 tsp	45
total calories:		265
Lunch (261 calories)		
bread	1 slice	73
skim milk	½ cup	40
tuna fish salad		
water-packed tuna fish	¼ cup	73
vegetables:		
one small carrot		
one small stalk celery		
one small tomato		
¼ medium cucumber		
lettuce		
¼ raw green pepper		
2 tbsp raw onion	(total for vegetables =)	50
apple	1 small	25
total calories:		261
Dinner (384 calories)		
lean pork chop	3 ounces	219
(without bone or fat)		
cauliflower	½ cup	25
macaroni	½ cup	70
salad:		
lettuce and		
4 radishes	as desired	0
tomatoes	½ cup	25
margarine	1 tsp	45
total calories:		384
Late night snack (75 calories)		
graham cracker	1 (2½ sq. in.)	35
grapes	12	40
total calories:		75

particular is so high that no one who must watch his weight can afford to consume these high caloric foods. Foods containing such excessive amounts of fats and carbohydrates will upset the diabetic's sugar and fat metabolism. In the future, when the food industries will be required to make more information available concerning ingredients, it will be possible to modify this list of "eat-nots". In the meantime, the diabetic should not take any chances with these foods and instead should select his foods from the list of substitute foods at the end of the book. The second of the following two tables and the recipe suggestions show the kind of menu plan best suited to the diabetic patient.

"eat-nots" — diet to lose weight

Since 90% of all diabetics are overweight and must lose weight to lower their blood sugar level, they are advised to adhere to the 1000 calorie diet. Diabetics belonging to the minority 10% of normal weight diabetics may of course double the number of calories suggested here.

Comparison of these two tables shows that the diet recommended for the diabetic contains more lean meat, vegetables, salads and fruits and much less fat and carbohydrates than the common American dishes listed in the first table. This emphasis on healthy foods rather than on processed foods permits the diabetic to calculate the exact nutritional content and caloric value, besides of course allowing him to adhere to a balanced and healthy diet. The method of substituting one food for another by using the substitute foods lists at the end of the book will be explained in detail later on. Table 3 is an example of food substitutions which can be made for the basic outline given in Table 2.

Recipe Suggestions

A housewife who cooks for a diabetic and healthy family members need not make any special preparations to follow the diabetes diet. We have used boldface type in the following recipes to emphasize the quantity which must be set aside for the diabetic. Although these recipes have been set up for four persons, adjustments in quantities can be made to prepare the meal for one, two or three persons.

sound nutrition for the entire family

The diabetic family member can easily participate in the family dinner, the one meal which requires greater preparation on the

45

part of the housewife. This is, of course, possible only if the family adheres to a healthy and well-balanced diet. A little extra effort then makes it possible to cook for the diabetic while also preparing the meal for the rest of the family.

Diabetic dinner #1

suggested meal #1

lean pork chops
cauliflower
potatoes
fresh strawberries

Ingredients for four persons (including one diabetic)

Lean pork chops;
4 lean pork chops each weighing 125 grams, pepper, 40 grams margarine, low fat broth.

Heat the margarine in a non-stick pan. Flatten the pork chops and brown them on both sides in the fat. Add pepper for taste and pour some low-fat broth over it. Allow the meat to cook for about ten minutes. Pour the meat juice over the pork chops while serving. **One pork chop with meat juice is for the diabetic.**

Cauliflower
one cauliflower weighing 800 to 1000 grams, water, margarine, herbs and spices.

Clean and wash the cauliflower and place in boiling salt water. Cook it for 20 to 30 minutes over low heat. Drain off water. Melt margarine and pour over cauliflower. ¼ **of cauliflower is for**

Potatoes
Peel and wash the potatoes, then cut them up and cook in salt water for about 20 minutes. Use a scale to determine the amount **for the diabetic, 195 grams.**

46

Fresh strawberries

Wash and prepare the strawberries (600 grams) and **set 150 grams aside for the diabetic.**

Nutritional value per person

Healthy person	Diabetic
Healthy person	**Diabetic**
35 grams protein	36 grams protein
28 grams fat	28 grams fat
55 grams carbohydrates	47 grams carbohydrates
629 calories	625 calories

Diabetic Dinner #2

suggested meal #2

roll-'em-ups
string beans
potatoes
stewed apricots

Ingredients for four persons (including one diabetic).

Roll-'em-ups

One pound round steak sliced into four slices of 125 grams each, pepper, mustard, four thin strips of bacon with fat removed, 2 dill pickles, 2 small potatoes, 2 small onions, paprika powder, 40 grams margarine, low-fat broth, 15 grams flour (not for diabetic).

Dry off each slice of steak and sprinkle with pepper, and coat with mustard. Cut dill pickles into strips. Wash tomatoes and cut them. Peel the onions and slice them. Place the bacon, dill pickle strips, half of the cut tomatoes, and onion slices on the thin slices of steak and sprinkle with paprika. Roll up each steak and fasten with toothpick or thread. Heat the margarine in a stewing pan and brown the rolled up steaks on all sides. Add the remaining tomatoes and onion slices and if desired another slice of dill pickle with mustard, and stew. Then fill pan with hot low-fat broth or water, and cook until tender for about 1½ hours. If necessary, add more liquid.

47

Take the roll-'em-ups out of the sauce when tender and pour the meat juice over them after passing it through a sieve. **One roll-'em-up is for the diabetic.** For the other family members, flour may be added to the meat juice to make gravy. If a special sauce thickener for diabetics is used, then the diabetic may also have gravy.

String beans

800 grams fresh string beans, basil or savory, water, salt, 40 grams margarine, parsley.

Wash and prepare string beans and put them in boiling salt water with the savory or basil. Cook until tender for 15 or 20 minutes. Drain the string beans. Serve with melted margarine, savory or basil and fresh chopped parsley. **¼ of the string beans are for the diabetic.**

Potatoes

Peel and wash the potatoes, cook until tender in salt water. **Set 195 grams aside for the diabetic.**

Stewed apricots

400 grams pitless apricots, artificial sweetener in liquid form.

Wash and cut the apricots in half, removing the pit. Bring water with 1 tsp artificial sweetner to boil and cook the apricots on medium heat until soft. To improve the flavor, cook the fruit with one of the pits. If necessary, add more artificial sweetener for the diabetic.

Nutritional value per person:

Healthy person
35 grams protein
27 grams fat
62 grams carbohydrate
652 calories

Diabetic
36 grams protein
27 grams fat
49 grams carbohydrate
636 calories

Diabetic dinner #3

Goulash with mushrooms
rice
salad
homemade sherbert

Ingredients for four persons (including one diabetic).

Goulash with mushrooms

500 grams lean beef, 60 grams margarine, pepper, paprika, one onion, low-fat broth, 20 grams sour cream (10% fat), 200 grams canned mushrooms.

Dry the beef and cut into uniform squares. Heat margarine in a non-stick pan, brown the meat on all sides and spice with salt, pepper, paprika and chopped onions. Add low-fat broth and cook until tender for about 60 minutes.

Drain mushrooms and add to goulash. Add sour cream and add more spices to make it hot and spicy. **¼ of goulash is for the diabetic.**

Rice

250 grams rice, water

Add rice to boiling salt water and cook, covered, for about 20 minutes over low heat until all water is absorbed. **About 150 grams of cooked rice is the diabetic's portion.** Tip: cook rice separately for the diabetic because rice can be made to absorb different amounts of water, usually 3 to 3½ times the raw rice.

Salad

One head of boston lettuce, parsley, basil, dill, chives, tarragon, 1½ tbsp. vegetable oil, lemon juice, liquid artificial sweetener

Clean and wash the lettuce and allow to drip dry. Finely chop the herbs. Mix the oil, lemon juice, some liquid artificial sweetener and the herbs. Pour the salad sauce over lettuce leaves and mix lightly. **¼ of salad is for the diabetic.**

49

Homemade raspberry sherbert

500 grams raspberries, three beaten eggwhites, juice from one lemon, two tablespoons liquid artificial sweetener

Wash the raspberries and mash with fork. Add artificial sweetener and lemon juice. Mix beaten eggwhites with mashed raspberries and freeze. Allow sherbert to soften for five minutes before serving. **One portion may be set aside for the diabetic.**

Nutritional value per person

Healthy person	Diabetic
39 grams protein	39 grams protein
24 grams fat	24 grams fat
50 grams carbohydrate	48 grams carbohydrate
629 calories	597 calories

Variety Using Substitutes

suit your personal taste

The diabetic is not required to eat only what has been suggested in Table 3. Instead, he should use the outline in Table 2 to determine the type and quantity of food he may eat. Each meal can then be adapted to the diabetic's taste and, with a bit of creativity, can be varied a great deal.

Substitutes are foods with the same value of carbohydrates, fats and proteins that can be substituted for one another. It is particularly important not to change the amount of carbohydrates when substituting foods.

All the products in the bread substitute list at the end of the book have the same amount of carbohydrates as one slice of bread, 15 grams. Please note that a large number of vegetables also fall into this category. When substituting one portion of one food in the list for another care must be taken to exchange the exact quantity specified. For example, the serving sizes equal to one slice of bread for some of the bread substitutes are the following:

½ english muffin
5 Triscuit crackers
½ cup macaroni
⅓ cup rice
⅓ cup lima beans
½ cup whipped potatoes
½ cup winter squash

Since the diabetic must pay attention to the speed with which carbohydrates are absorbed, he should be careful to substitute foods within the same category. For example, he should exchange one fruit for another or one carbohydrate-rich vegetable for another (for example, ½ bagel for 1 slice rye bread).

We would now like to give two examples to clarify the system of exchanging one food for another. The diet plan outlined in Table 2 specifies that the diabetic on a 1000 calorie diet may consume one bread substitute for breakfast. In the example in Table 3, we substituted one slice of toast. However, the diabetic may also substitute ½ english muffin or ¾ cup dry cereal for this one bread exchange. The diabetic on this diet may not eat a whole english muffin because this would be equal to two bread substitutes as can be seen from the list.

The second example is from the dinner outlined in Table 2. The diabetic on this diet plan sees that he may again consume one bread substitute. If the diabetic likes biscuits with dinner, then he may eat one 2 inch biscuit. However, if he prefers macaroni, then he may have ½ cup, or if he would rather eat corn, then he may have ⅓ cup, or else ½ cup of green cooked peas. Each of these portions has the nutritional value of 15 grams carbohydrates and 2-2.5 grams protein. Each portion listed under bread substitutions supplies 70 calories.

There is also an exchange list for fats. This list should be consulted like the list for bread exchange to bring variety into the menu plan.

caution:
hidden fats!

Substitutions for the fat exchanges listed in the diet plan outlined in Table 2 must be made with great care because the invisible fats contained in meat, sausage, milk, and milk products must also be taken into account. It is best to use only ⅓ to ½ of the fat substitute to spread on toast or for cooking. Foods rich in protein must be exchanged with care because the fat content of these foods varies and must not exceed the amount specified in the diet. Foods which contain many grams of fat also are high in calorie count. Moreover, saturated fats (animal fats) should be avoided for other health reasons.

In contrast to the bread and fat substitutes which must always be carefully calculated, the foods rich in protein but low in carbohydrates and fats may be exchanged liberally. Only those diabetics who suffer from a severe kidney problem have to restrict the protein intake.

The diabetic can adhere to a diet plan which specifies substitutes only if he carefully weighs all his foods. The diabetic should always use a scale to determine the exact number of grams. Since most kitchen scales are not so precise, the diabetic should use a special scale for diet purposes. (You may be more used to measuring in pounds and ounces but metric measurement—grams, etc.—is far simpler and, therefore, for practical purposes, more accurate.) To measure fluids, the diabetic should use measuring cups which specify grams and milliliters. Diet scales and measuring cups are indispensable for the diabetic kitchen. Other measuring devices may also be used. Before using spoons, (teaspoons, tablespoons or scoops) cups or other utensils, the scales should be used to determine how many grams or cubic centimeters each contains. The diabetic may use these utensils instead of the scales if he knows how much they hold.

With practice, one quickly learns to judge exact quantities in a reliable manner just by looking at the food. This, however, does not mean that the diabetic may rely only on visual judgment to weigh ingredients, because subjective elements such as desire

use a diet scale

learn to use your eye for weighing

Frequently-used measurements

Utensil	examples
one level teaspoon	10 grams of diabetic marmalade
	5 grams flour
	5 grams milk
	2 grams oil
	2 grams red wine
	8-10 grams butter
	8-10 grams margarine
one level tablespoon	20 grams margarine
	10 grams cream
	15 grams milk
one cup	125 grams (cc.)
one water glass	150-200 grams (cc.)
one soup bowl	¼ liter

52

and appetite may influence this judgment. The diabetic should use his diet scale to control his ability to determine the quantity from time to time.

Artificial Sweeteners

substituting for sweet things

Although the diabetic should avoid sugar, he need not give up sweet things completely. Not all foods which taste sweet are excluded from the diabetic diet. Artificial sweeteners and sugar substitutes play an important role becuase he may use these instead of the usual sugar (cane sugar and brown sugar).

sugar substi-
tutes contain
carbohydrates

Although sugar substitutes belong to the category of carbohydrates, they are digested more slowly and independently of insulin up to a certain amount. Most sugar substitutes contain saccharin. The calorie count of these sugar substitutes is indicated on the package and must be taken into consideration when the daily carbohydrate allowance is calculated. Large amounts of sugar substitutes may have a negative influence on sugar metabolism.

are artificial
sweeteners
harmful?

Artificial sweeteners are synthetic products which have no calories and may be used to sweeten foods. The most important chemical substances are saccharin and cyclamates. Products using saccharin are 400-500 times as sweet as the regular household sugar. Artificial sweeteners containing cyclamates are 35 times as sweet as household sugar and products which contain both saccharin and cyclamates are about 90 times as sweet as regular sugar. In the U.S., the Food and Drug Administration removed cyclamates from the market, claiming that this chemical caused bladder cancer in laboratory animals. After certain studies showed that massive doses of saccharin could also cause cancer in laboratory animals, the FDA proposed a total ban on saccharins as well, but later settled for a label indicating the potential health hazard to laboratory animals. The possible carcinogenic effect of saccharin is generally considered to be less of a risk than the elevated blood sugar levels resulting from sugar intake. Almost all artificial sugars are soluble, can be cooked and baked without changing their chemical composition, and do not contain any calories in contrast to the sugar substitutes. They are particularly important for obese diabetics. Artificial sweeteners and sugar substitutes play an important role, for use not only in the diabetic's home but also in processed foods. Special products made for diabetics, such as good-tasting (remember to count calories!) jam show how useful these sugar substitutes can be.

A Tasty and Spicy Diet.

Diabetics are encouraged to season their food to bring out its flavor. Just like all other persons, diabetics are advised not to spice their foods excessively. The proper combination of one or two herbs or spices will make a dish taste better than the indiscriminate use of many different spices. Directions given in cookbooks show that the quantity of spices used is very important; in fact, one could speak of an "art" of seasoning. Spices should bring out the natural taste of food, rather than overpower it. Moreover, seasonings which have opposite effects and tastes should not be used in combination, since they then cancel each other out.

the art of seasoning

Since there is such a large variety of herbs and spices, we can only enumerate a few of them.

Fresh or dried herbs may be used. Many of them can be grown in a garden or flower box.

Herbs

For example:

Basil, bay, burnett, caroway, shefril, chives, coriander, dill, fennil, marjoram, mint, oregano, parsley, rosemary, sage, savory, tarragon, thyme.

Spices

For example: allspice, cayenne, cinnamon, cloves, curry, dry mustard, ginger root, lemon verbena, lime, mace, mint essence, nutmeg, paprika, pepper, saffron, shallot, tumeric, vanilla.

Ground spices lose their taste if cooked with the food. Exceptions to this general rule are curry, chili and paprika, which should be cooked with the food to develop their taste. Most spices must be added to the food right after cooking and other seasonings may be added at the table.

Fresh herbs should be truly fresh. They can be preserved in a glass of water overnight in the refrigerator, or may be stored in the freezer after being chopped up. In contrast to most fresh herbs which should not be cooked with the food, dried herbs develop their flavor only if they are cooked. If a meal is being cooked with foods which require little preparation, then the dry herbs used for seasoning should be allowed to stand in a little water to develop their taste before adding them to the food.

how much salt may I use?

Salt brings out the natural taste of food by making it fuller or rounding it off. However, the use of salt for diabetics is often restricted or forbidden completely because the diabetic may suffer from a weak heart, kidney problems, or hypertension. Since most foods naturally contain salt, these diabetics must avoid salty foods and adding salt either in the kitchen or at the table. These patients should learn to cook with herbs and spices only.

One must enjoy the taste of onions and garlic to use them freely. Many consider garlic and onions to be especially "healthy". Garlic in particular is so potent that each must make his own decision to use it.

vinegar and mustard

Many dishes do not taste the way they should unless a dab of mustard or some vinegar is added. Fermented vinegar is made from alcohol (beer, wine, brandy), fruit or malt; seasoned vinegar is made with added tarragon, basil or garlic. Various kinds of mustard are available, ranging from sharp to almost sweet. A diabetic who likes to use large amounts of mustard should remember that it contains sugar and starches (the exact amounts are usually unknown).

Pickles, tomatoes, radishes and spring onions are not included in the list of spices or herbs. Nonetheless, these vegetables may be used to add flavor to food and are particularly suited for the calorie-conscious diabetic since they contain few calories and carbohydrates.

using cheese to season

Certain kinds of cheese may also be used to season food. Cheese is an important spice if its special flavor is considered. Spicy cheeses include parmesan, green cheese, goat cheese, and sharp cheddar. Since cheese may lose its aroma quickly, it should always be grated freshly. Diabetics, however, must be careful in their use of spicy cheeses because they generally contain large amounts of fats, calories and salt.

Finally, beverages may also be used to marinate and flavor food or else to serve a dish flambé. Here again, the diabetic must restrict his use. Many of the alcoholic beverages suggested for seasoning food are rich in calories or carbohydrates. Recommended for spicing are natural rums, wine and cognac.

Dining Out

The diabetic must know how much he can eat and drink before he may dine out. With this knowledge, he will not have any difficulty choosing the proper meals in restaurants. If invited to someone's home for dinner, he can determine which dishes are permitted without offending his host. To avoid upsetting the metabolism, he should not follow the encouragement of the host to "have a little more."

The diabetic should keep his diet in mind when he chooses his vacation spot. Naturally, resorts which offer hotels or boarding houses with dietary kitchens for diabetics are highly recommended.

If the resort does not offer any special dietary kitchen, then the diabetic will find it less difficult to adhere to the diet if he chooses his dishes from a menu than if he receives three meals per day as part of a package deal. Of course, he will have even less difficulty if he vacations in a place offering a kitchenette.

Beverages and the Diabetes Diet

milk in the right quantity

The diabetic should apply the same guidelines to his choice of beverages as to the choice of foods. If the beverages do not contain any calories, then the diabetic may drink any quantity he desires. However, the diabetic must restrict consumption of certain beverages and must avoid others altogether. Milk occupies a special position. Since milk contains carbohydrates, fats, proteins and calories, as well as calcium and vitamins, the diabetic should drink milk to balance his diet. If the diabetic carefully calculates the calorie count and fat content (8 ounces — ¼ liter — contains 9 grams fat), then he may drink up to 8 ounces (¼ liter) per day.

Skim milk contains *everything* except fat. The diabetic should choose skim milk products if he is on a reducing diet. When choosing yogurt, the diabetic must carefully distinguish yogurt made from whole milk from that made with skim milk (only the skim milk yogurt is low-fat).

Lemonades, soft drinks like Coca-cola, and other beverages containing a large amount of sugar (fruit-flavored drinks), as well as frozen concentrated juices are not suited for the diabetic because they contain a large amount of carbohydrates which are quickly absorbed. However, the diabetic may drink unsweetened, freshly pressed juices in small calculated amounts, if he takes the calorie content into account.

caution with
fruit juices!

Beverages

No restriction:
> water and non-caloric soft drinks
> mineral water
> coffee and tea without milk and sugar

Restricted, quantity must be calculated:
> milk (all kinds)
> yogurt (all kinds)
> freshly pressed fruit juices
> diet fruit juices
> diet frozen concentrated juices
> diet lemonade
> diet wine
> diet champagne
> diet beer
> brandy, cognac, whiskey

Not allowed
> fruit juices
> frozen concentrated juices
> lemonade
> soft drinks
> sweet wines
> liqueur
> regular champagne
> beer (all regular kinds)
> sweetened cocktails

Diet drinks contain a very small amount of, or no carbohydrates. Some artificially sweetened beverages have so few
calories that the diabetic does not need to take them into
account. He may drink these as desired. However, most diet fruit
juices, diet beers and diet champagnes contain a small number
of calories which must be calculated into the diet.

beverages
have calories

Are Alcohol, Coffee, Tea and Tobacco Allowed?

The role of alcoholic beverages in the diabetes diet is often
misunderstood. Some patients avoid alcohol completely. Others
believe that certain alcoholic beverages have a beneficial effect
on their sugar metabolism.

It must of course be said that alcohol is not particularly healthy
for the diabetic or for anyone else. Nonetheless, alcoholic

Caloric content of alcoholic beverages

Type of beverage	Quantity	Cal
*Regular malt liquors	1 small glass (0.2 l)	114
Diabetic diet beer	1 bottle (.3 l)	135
Brandy (76 proof)	1 glass (2 ml)	49
Gin	1 glass (2 ml)	37
Whiskey	1 glass (4 ml)	100
Rum (90 proof)	1 glass (2 ml)	49
*Vermouth (42 proof)	1 glass (5 ml)	57
*Port wine	1 glass (5 ml)	70
*Sherry	1 glass (5 ml)	55
White wine	1 glass (⅛ ml)	75
Red wine	1 glass (⅛ ml)	83
Hard cider	1 glass (¼ ml)	113
*Regular champagne	1 glass (8 ml)	67
Diet champagne	1 glass (8 ml)	56

*denotes alcoholic beverages the diabetic may not
consume due to their high carbohydrate content.

alcohol
allowed in
proper
quantity

beverages play an important part in our life-styles. The diabetic may enjoy small quantities of alcoholic beverages which have only a small or no influence on his carbohydrate metabolism, if he carefully calculates their effect on his metabolic condition.

The following alcoholic beverages are not permitted because of their high carbohydrate content: liqueur, sweet brandies, sweetened cocktails, all sweet (not dry) white and red wines, champagne and regular beer of any type.

Since one ounce of alcohol contains about 57 calories (one gram = 7 calories) alcohol provides a large quantity of energy. As a result, the weight-conscious diabetic may consume only small quantities of alcoholic beverages even if they contain few or no carbohydrates. The alcoholic beverages in this category include brandy, cognac, whiskey, gin, rum, and cordials. If the diabetic is invited to have a drink at a reception, before a dinner or at a party, then he should choose a very small amount of whiskey with lots of soda water and ice.

caution:
sweet wines

Wines which contain less than 4 grams of sugar per liter and less than 12% alcohol do not have a decisive influence on the sugar metabolism. Obese diabetics, however, must restrict their consumption of these wines due to their high caloric content. The diabetic should be equally critical toward unsweetened fermented fruit juices such as hard cider.

Certain diabetics must take three factors into consideration. 1. Some diabetics simply cannot "hold their liquor." 2. Other diabetics who must take oral hypoglycemic agents react more quickly to alcohol and are intoxicated after only a small amount. 3. Diabetics develop liver damage more easily than healthy persons. Any diabetic whose liver is already damaged should avoid alcohol. Of course, diabetics and healthy persons alike should not drink alcohol if they must drive.

alcohol and
medication

Alcoholic beverages must figure in the diet plan. An obese diabetic in particular must consume a smaller quantity of food if he wants to enjoy alcoholic beverages. The diabetic should calculate the number of calories in the alcohol and then restrict his intake of carbohydrates, fats and proteins to equal this amount. He should not simply exclude all carbohydrates (bread or fruit) from his meal plan for that particular day.

coffee and
tea are
allowed

Other beverages which may have a stimulating effect are coffee and tea. The caffeine contained in coffee, as well as in tea

59

— when taken in larger amounts — has a stimulating effect. The diabetic need not restrict his tea and coffee consumption.

smoking is harmful

An entire book should be devoted to the topic of nicotine. It must be made perfectly clear that nicotine is poison for the blood vessels. Damage due to smoking is found particularly in the heart, the large blood vessels in the pelvis and the legs, as well as in the bronchi and the lungs. The consequences of smoking include heart attack, "smoker's leg", bronchitis and lung cancer. The blood vessel damage quickly adds up in diabetics who smoke. Diabetes in itself is a risk factor for vascular diseases, but when the damaging effect of nicotine is added, then the incidence of vascular damage is increased. Recent medical studies indicate that smoking promotes the development of eye damage found in diabetics. If you are a diabetic and still smoke, you should under all circumstances try to "kick the habit." A non-smoker should not begin to smoke. The challenge for the smoker to give up smoking is often difficult to meet. However difficult it may seem, it is possible to quit smoking. Millions of Americans have done so already.

Economical Choice of Groceries

how to avoid excessive costs

The diabetic probably leads a more expensive life than a healthy person because he must buy a higher precentage of high-priced food rich in potein (lean meat, fish and poultry), as well as more vegetables and fresh fruits. These added expenses can, however, be controlled.

The diabetic can save a lot of money by carefully shopping for groceries. Although lean meat is generally far more expensive than fatty meat, the diabetic may not have to pay more if he watches for specials. He can take advantage of a special offer by buying large quantities and storing these in his freezer. When buying vegetables, one should buy those which are in season. Moreover, the diabetic should choose low-fat cheeses which are less expensive, rather than an expensive French cheese (which may also contain too much fat). In this manner one may compensate for the inevitably higher cost of groceries.

Other greater expenses, which cannot be avoided, include the cost of diet foods such as dietary sugar, dietary marmalade and diet juices. However, in the case of other groceries, the diabetic may chose common foods and may be able to save money by preparing juices and jams himself.

It may prove just as expensive to fail to bring the urinary and blood sugar under control. Weight gain is not only unnecessary and harmful, but also entails a higher cost for groceries. Persons who eat more than they should must of course pay more than they like.

Essentials for the Diabetic's Kitchen

In discussing the diabetes diet we have referred to numerous useful utensils. What should the diabetic have in his kitchen?

Absolutely essential reference material

- diet plan
- exchange lists

Absolutely essential utensils

- a diet scale showing gram determinations
- various measuring cups showing grams (g.), cubic centimeters (ccm.) or milliliters (ml.) to be measured
- other common utensils for which exact quantity can be determined (spoons, beakers, cups, etc.)

Recommended utensils

- non-stick pots and pans
- casserole dishes
- aluminum foil
- roasting bags
- grill
- pressure cooker

7. Weight Reduction for the Obese Diabetic

The most important treatment measure for the obese adult diabetic is weight reduction. Obesity promotes not only metabolic disorders — the blood sugar level cannot easily be controlled without normal weight — but also the development of other risk-factors: disorders of fat metabolism, high blood pressure and elevated uric acid (and together with this, gout). The ideal goal is the ideal weight:

Ideal weight for women = normal weight minus 15%.
Ideal weight for men = normal weight minus 10%.

Wrong Ideas and Pseudo-Alibis

We must confront some wrong ideas and alibis which may be used as an excuse to avoid weight reduction. For example, many believe in a genetic disorder that "has always been in our family." Obesity cannot be inherited. What the family does transmit are normal but incorrect eating habits. Grandmother was a good cook and believed like all other family members now do that "good eating keeps body and soul together!"

self-delusion

One often hears: "I have heavy bones!" Actually, the entire skeleton weighs an average of 18 to 22 pounds (8 to 10 kilograms) in large people.

Many think "I use up all the food I eat!" and may have some right to make this assertion, although scientists have not yet been able to prove differences in energy consumption. What is certain is that one will gain weight if one consumes dispro-portionately large amounts of food and that one can lose weight only if one eats and drinks less than one requires.

pseudo-alibi "glands"

Many of those who are overweight presume that a disease causes their obesity: "My glands are causing my problem!" This excuse is valid in very rare cases, actually in no more than 0.1%. Glandular or endocrinologic disorders would be recognized the moment they appear, since they cause serious and obvious

62

problems. A snide response to this "excuse" is that, of course, there is a gland involved here: the salivary gland!

do you perform heavy physical activity?

Others explain their craving for food by saying that "if one works, one must eat!" In our modern world, few people exert themselves physically. Heavy physical activity is not necessary due to mechanization. Since few of us exert ourselves physically we need a small number of calories to maintain weight.

fat from eating too much

"I really don't eat that much" is surely the most frequent excuse. If you believe this, you may be correct at the present moment. If you ate too much in earlier years and gained weight, then your body does not require as much as earlier to maintain the long-term obesity. People using this excuse, however, often forget that they consume calories when drinking. Moreover, even small amounts of calories lead to a clear gain in weight if consumed regularly in addition to the regular meals.

If you are afraid that you exercise less than you should, you are probably right. However, lack of exercise is not sufficient to explain obesity. It takes quite a lot of exercise to rid oneself of the caloric content of only one glass of beer (120 calories).

Daily stress does not lead to calorie loss, though many may complain about stress. An adult male working in an office consumes only about 1000 calories in the course of a day.

Weight Reduction through Behavior Modification

change your eating habits

In recent years, psychologists specializing in behavior modification have performed many studies concerning eating behavior, appetite and satiation in obese and normal weight persons. These studies show that the slender subject obeys inner signals of satiation and stops eating when satiated, thus avoiding overeating. Whereas slender persons lose appetite as they achieve satiation, obese persons experience increased appetite while eating. For these persons, the saying "appetite is developed while eating" holds true. Obese persons are stimulated by the appeal of food even when satiated. Their appetite is stronger than the feeling of satiation. Since they lack an inner regulatory mechanism for satiation they do not stop eating when they should.

Since the obese patient cannot orient himself by inner regulatory mechanisms, he must learn to orient himself by outside indicators to lose weight. These outside indicators can vary a great deal, but they all serve the same purpose of behavior modification. A behaviorist, Dr. Pudel, has composed a list of principles to guide the obese patient:

1. At home, I will eat only at places and times I have established.
2. When I eat, I will only eat and drink and will not turn on the television or radio.
3. I will complete the preparation of each meal before I begin to eat. I will put away all remaining ingredients. Only then will I begin to eat.
4. After each meal I will immediately clear off all dishes and leftovers.
5. I will not leave any foods or drinks standing around my apartment.
6. Before going to the grocery store, I will make up a grocery list.
7. In the store I will buy only what is on my list.
8. I will go grocery shopping only if I have already eaten or am not hungry.
9. Before taking a bite of food I will divide it in half one more time.
10. I will chew each bite of food at least twenty times while counting and consciously tasting it. While chewing I will put down my knife and fork.
11. I will spend at least 20 minutes eating my main meals.
12. I will keep beverages and soups on my tongue until I have counted to ten. After each sip I will put my glass back down on the table.
13. I will make a pause for one to two minutes at the half-way point of each meal.
14. I will leave some food on the plate after each meal.
15. I will never snack between meals, as, for example, while grocery shopping, preparing meals in the kitchen, before going to bed, or out of sheer boredom.
16. Before being invited to dinner, I will decide exactly what I will eat and drink. While dining out I will divide my portions of food so that I will always have something to eat.

A close reading of these behavior rules for the obese shows that the obese patient must learn to eat and drink only under certain predetermined conditions (rules 1 through 3), that he should try to reduce and control the temptation of food in his surroundings (rules 4 through 8), that he should try to make a habit of eating slowly and therefore less (rules 9 through 13), and that he should determine his strategy before beginning a meal or before encountering situations which may cause problems, for example, when invited to dine out (rules 14 through 16).

Success with the Weight Reduction Plan for Diabetics

The diet plan for the obese adult diabetic is based on a weight reduction plan. This is a balanced diet composed of different kinds of foodstuffs which have less calories and which as a whole are highly beneficial for the obese diabetic.

In addition to this balanced diet which contains all necessary nutrients in the proper amounts, there is a large number of dietary recommendations for diabetics which were established long ago and have been revised repeatedly. All these recommendations can lead to weight loss if less calories are consumed than are needed. Unusual or extreme diets do not make the most important thing possible: an effective and permanent modification of behavior, a change of life-style. Some of these diets may even damage the health of the individual because they include no or few carbohydrates. They may be used *temporarily* by adult diabetics, as has been shown by some specialists, but the best diet for such a person is a balanced diet with a reduced number of calories (the weight reduction plan for diabetics). Of course, the diabetic must consume all the necessary nutrients in the proper quantities. The slogan "eat sensibly" should be kept in mind by the obese adult diabetic for whom the reduced diet is certainly the best way of losing weight.

8. Long-Term Drug Therapy

The diabetes diet combined with weight reduction and physical activity reduces the burden on the pancreas. In the case of relative insulin deficiency in particular, the obese adult diabetic will need less insulin as soon as he loses weight. Should insulin deficiency remain significant when he has reached his normal weight, then he must rely on oral hypoglycemic agents or on insulin injections.

Possible methods of treating insulin deficiency

- Diet, weight reduction, physical activity to relieve the overburdened insulin production.
- Intake of the blood sugar lowering sulfonylurea tablets to stimulate insulin production.
- Injections of insulin to replace amounts lacking.
- Oral biquanide tablets to make the available insulin more effective is no longer permitted in the U.S.

Treatment with Oral Hypoglycemic Agents

tablets stimulate the pancreas

Many diabetics can treat their disease with oral hypoglycemic agents and diet. Prerequisite for successful treatment with oral agents is that the pancreas be able to produce a certain amount of insulin. Therefore, pills that lower blood sugar have an effect only in adult diabetics with a relative insulin deficiency.

The so-called sulfonylurea compounds stimulate the pancreas to excrete insulin. Continuous research of the pharmaceutical companies has enabled them to offer a large variety of sulfonylurea compounds which lower blood sugar. Today, many different kinds of these pills are available. Drugs developed within the last 10 years are usually prescribed. These pills are to be taken either in the morning or else in the morning and the evening with meals (in contrast to the other pills which must be taken three times per day.) The physician will write out the proper prescription taking the individual metabolic disorders as well as the effectiveness of each tablet into consideration.

Sulfonylurea compounds to lower blood sugar

trade name	size of pill	usual daily dose
orinase	500 mg.	500-2000 mg.
tolinase	100-250 mg.	100-1000 mg.
diabinese	100-250 mg.	100-500 mg.
dymelor	250-500 mg.	250-1500 mg.

adhere to the prescription

The efficacy of sulfonylurea compounds is not enhanced if the daily dosage is increased beyond the maximum indicated. A higher dosage of tablets will not lower the blood sugar level any further.

Another group of so-called oral anti-diabetics is the biquanides. Since rare but serious side effects were discovered recently resulting from this group of drugs, physicians no longer prescribe them in the U.S. (By order of the FDA, biquanides are not available for general use in the U.S.)

The mechanism of action of the biquanides is not yet understood. It is known that they help make the available insulin more effective, but do not stimulate the pancreas to release more insulin as the sulfonylurea compunds do. In the past, biquanides were prescribed if the diet and sulfonylurea drugs were not sufficient in the treatment.

Side Effects of Oral Hypoglycemic Agents

Any effective medication sometimes causes side effects. This also holds true for anti-diabetics although side effects are only *rarely* observed.

side-effects are rare

The side effects typical for most drugs are rarely found in the case of the sulfonylurea compounds: changes in the white blood count and differential blood count, allergic reactions, and stomach and intestinal disorders.

In 1970, an American study was published which generated great interest and provoked a discussion still continuing today. It showed that the sulfonylurea and biquanide compounds elevate the risk of development of heart and blood vessel complications. Other researchers were not able to confirm these observations.

67

Many studies contradicted the American results. For this reason, treatment with oral hypoglycemic agents has not been abandoned. After this medical dispute, physicians stressed the basics of any treatment of diabetes, proper nutrition and normalization of body weight, more than ever before.

Hypoglycemia, decreased blood sugar level, is strictly speaking not a side effect of the sulfonylurea compounds, but a sign that they are almost too effective. Hypoglycemia results only when the blood sugar is lowered too much, thus making the desired effect of the oral hypoglycemic agent (necessary blood sugar lowering) into a side effect (hypoglycemia).

mistakes and their consequences

There is a risk of hypoglycemia when a diabetic who could be treated with diet alone also takes oral hypoglycemic agents. But even diabetics who actually need to take these oral agents may be affected by hypoglycemia, if they forget to consume a meal or take too many pills, or experience unusual physical activity.

Hypoglycemia resulting from sulfonylurea usually develops gradually after several hours but it can be particularly severe. The physician must be consulted immediately because hypoglycemia may linger on for quite a while and also because the physician must reexamine the methods of treatment employed up to that time.

if other drugs are taken at the same time

Sometimes hypoglycemia is the result of the combined effect of the sulfonylurea compounds and other medication which must be taken and which also has a certain blood sugar lowering effect. One example of such a drug is the medication taken for rheumatism. Some of the earlier sulfonylurea compounds are not compatible with the drinking of alcohol. Pregnant women should not take these drugs because it is not yet absolutely clear whether these oral agents damage the fetus.

biquanide compounds

The biquanides cause disturbances and complaints more frequently than sulfonylurea compounds (loss of appetite, a pasty or metallic taste in the mouth, nausea, a feeling of pressure in the abdomen, vomiting and diarrhea). The one dangerous side effect of the biquanides, lactic acidosis (an excess of lactic acid), is rare, but when it does occur it is fatal, and this actually led to the FDA decision to remove the drug.

Since biquanides are no longer available for general use, physicians again emphasize diet. This new emphasis on diet resulted from the discovery of an additional side effect of the treatment with oral hypoglycemic agents: diabetics tend to neglect their diet because they believe that the oral agent is sufficient to control blood sugar.

Diet and Oral Hypoglycemic Agents

Treatment with oral hypoglycemic agents is probably the simplest long-term treatment method, especially when compared to the demand that the diabetic adhere to a strict diet. Some may unconsciously hope their diabetes will disappear when they take two or three pills a day. This hope is deceptive; the patient must understand that the diet is the basis for any diabetic treatment. No treatment can be successful if it does not include diet.

We repeat: treatment with sulfonylureas can be effective only when combined with proper diet. Pills should be taken only when good diabetes control cannot be achieved by a proper diet alone. Of course, the obesity of a diabetic shows his failure to follow the dietary rules as long as he is overweight. Sometimes temporarily normal values of blood sugar can be achieved by simply using the oral agents. However, the blood sugar cannot permanently be controlled and the risks of obesity cannot be avoided as long as the patient is overweight.

Such criticism of oral hypoglycemic agents is certainly necessary from time to time, yet it is also important to realize what a great blessing these oral agents can be. These have made it possible for a large number of previously insulin dependent diabetics to switch to pills while remaining on a strict diet. The diabetic who can profit from the combined treatment of diet and pills today can hardly imagine the excitement among diabetics when pills were first introduced. But he will also be aware that these pills do not make the diet unnecessary, as was first hoped 25 years ago.

Sometimes diabetics make a vain attempt to correct dietary errors by using pills. But the negative effect of consuming a piece of cake cannot be corrected by simply taking an additional pill beyond the recommended daily dose. A diabetic treated with diet and oral hypoglycemic agents must adhere to both aspects of the treatment.

The experience with oral hypoglycemic agents over the past 25 years has shown that the effectiveness of such treatment declines after a number of years. For this reason, the blood sugar values of a diabetic may be elevated despite the stimulation of these pills. This shows that the release and production of insulin by the pancreas is slowly declining. These patients can then easily switch to insulin treatment. The insulin injections will ensure that the metabolism is brought under control.

Administration of Insulin

Patients whose pancreas produces no insulin or only minute amounts must be treated with insulin. This group of patients includes diabetics with juvenile and, to a lesser extent, maturity onset diabetes who do not react to treatment with oral hypo-glycemic agents. Treatment with insulin may also become

when tablets are no longer sufficient

necessary in certain temporary situations (which may become permanent) as for example after the patient has a coma, in pregnant diabetics who cannot be treated with diet alone, or finally in patients who are usually treated by pills but whose metabolism is subjected to the stress of an operation, an illness with fever or an accident.

Insulin is a protein taken from animal tissue (cattle and pigs). Insulin is usually packaged in 10 ml. vials which equals 10 cubic centimeters (cc). Since one cubic centimeter equals 40 units, one vial contains 400 units of insulin.

what are insulin units?

Insulin is measured in units. The average daily consumption in a normal adult is about 40 units. It must be injected and cannot be taken orally because it would be destroyed by the process of digestion.

Insulin for each individual requirement

There are various types of insulin which differ in their origin, composition and effectiveness. This large variety helps the physician find the insulin best suited to the individual's metabolism.

The so-called crystalline or regular insulins are fast-acting. They become effective shortly after injection, but are charac-terized by the short duration of effect. Fast-acting insulins are used almost exclusively in special situations, as a temporary measure when the blood sugar is being normalized for the first

70

time, during and after operations or after a child delivery, in the diabetic coma or in situations where metabolism is particularly variable. This type of insulin must be injected several times per day and always before a meal.

The intermediate-acting insulins are also called isophane or NPH (neutral protein Hagedorn and Lente). Certain materials have been added to insulin to prolong its action (for example, protein, zinc and globin) or by producing them by a certain method (crystallization). These are the most commonly used insulins and must ususally be injected twice a day about 30 minutes prior to a meal. The duration and peak of action vary from one patient to the next and depend on the injection site, the quantity of insulin and the speed of absorption from the subcutaneous fatty tissue.

Insulins of prolonged duration are effective from 24 to 36 hours. They are actually suited only to those patients who have a stable and balanced metabolism and who also lead a regular life. It is certainly more pleasant to inject insulin only once a day, between 30 and 90 minutes prior to breakfast, but it is difficult to properly control the blood sugar level with this type of insulin.

When the physician prescribes a certain kind of insulin for his patient, he considers not only its effectiveness, but also the metabolism and daily routine of the individual. Each patient must inject himself with the insulin best suited to his case.

If you require insulin, you should learn to inject it yourself. A patient is often admitted to a hospital to teach him how to inject insulin and to monitor possible side effects when the diabetic first uses it. You should not only learn how to inject insulin properly, but should also experience hypoglycemia, the most important side effect of treatment, in order to know what this means and what measures are to be taken. The diabetic may also be treated in outpatient care when first exposed to insulin, where he can consult his physician regularly and learn to inject insulin in the presence of the doctor.

Insulin injections and paraphernalia

As a diabetic you will have your own insulin, which may be either clear or cloudy in appearance. Clear insulin may be injected immediately, but cloudy insulin must be shaken before the

71

injection. The label on the bottle indicates the expiration date. Insulin is quite stable but can usually be used for only 2 to 3 years. It can be kept in a cool area, in the vegetable drawer in a refrigerator above 40°F — 4°C), or at room temperature. Insulin should not be subjected to extreme heat or cold.

Various types of needles and syringes are available today for insulin injection. Reusable syringes and stainless steel needles are frequently used. The size of the syringe depends upon the quantity of insulin which must be injected. The measurement in cubic centimeters is printed on the syringe barrel and usually corresponds to 40 units of insulin. The subdivisions on the barrel may indicate measurements in increments of .1 ml or in units of insulin. A subdivision of .1 ml equals about 4 units of insulin. For this reason, the quantities prescribed are usually multiples of 4, that is 4, 8, 12, 16 or 20 units. Syringes with special subdivisions or plastic syringes may also make it possible to measure intermediate quantities precisely.

The supplies used with reusable syringes and stainless steel needles include:

  2 reusable syringes
 12 hypodermic needles (either long = 14 mm or
    short = 11 mm)
  1 chromium-plated metal vial for storage
    (the most practical is cylindrical with a screw top)
  1 pair of tweezers
    cotton or alcohol swabs
    alcohol for disinfection
  1 sauce pan with stainless steel sieve.

If one uses disposable syringes, which are increasingly popular, one needs only extra needles, cotton or alcohol swabs, and alcohol for disinfection. The disposable needles may be obtained separately or may already be attached to the syringe. They are packaged in sterile plastic or paper covers and must be removed before use. Although disposable needles and syringes are intended to be used only once, experience has shown that they can sometimes be used more than once.

Recommended are disposable syringes with a long slender barrel, a plunger which can be seen clearly through the barrel, and a scale which is easily read. Syringes which have different markings on them are not recommended because they may be confusing. Of course, the syringes and plungers must be kept sterile. Plungers on disposable syringes must be cleaned of the last drops of insulin and be stored in a clean place. The needle must be replaced in the original protective cover. Reusable syringes must be disassembled to be cleaned and boiled for 10 minutes with needles and tweezers in a stainless steel sieve and sauce pan reserved for this purpose. Distilled water can be bought in a drug store or derived by boiling tap water for 15 minutes. The glass barrel may burst if placed directly in boiling water.

sterilizing reusable syringes

After the syringes are boiled and cooled, they are assembled and stored in the containers which have also been sterilized, without adding alcohol. The separate components of the syringe and needles should be handled with care, removed from the sieve with tweezers without touching the nozzle or needle at its tip. If the patient accidentally touches the needle or if it touches other objects, then these parts must be sterilized again.

If you carefully sterilize your supplies in this manner, then the process must be repeated only once a week or every two weeks. You may reuse your syringe and needles without any further cleaning. Although it should be self-evident, we must emphasize that each diabetic should use his own individual syringe. It is dangerous to loan your syringe to another person for injection, because hepatitis could be transmitted.

don't use another's syringe

Drawing up insulin

You must wash your hands carefully before taking the syringe and vial into your hands. The skin area where the injection will be made should be cleaned; a regular shower is sufficient. The additional disinfection with alcohol is then not generally necessary (although many clinics and physicians insist on it).

The same needle is used for drawing the insulin into the syringe and for the injection. It must first be attached to the barrel. Then draw the plunger until the syringe contains as much air as insulin to be withdrawn. Keeping the plunger in this position, insert the needle through the diaphragm top of the vial which is still standing upright, in such a way that the needle tip is

drawing up of insulin

located in the top the upper part of which contains air. Then push the air in the syringe into the vial in order to create pressure. This makes it possible to draw up the insulin without creating foam in the solution. Then invert the vial so that the needle points vertically to the top in the vial, and draw insulin into the syringe by pulling back the plunger. It is advisable to draw a few more units of insulin than is necessary. While continuing to hold the vial in the inverted position, you can now expel the air in the syringe into the bottle and push the extra amount of insulin back into the bottle until the exact desired amount of insulin is in the syringe.

injecting a mixture of insulin

The same general principle is applied when it is sometimes necessary to mix two different kinds of insulin. Care must be taken not to inject a small amount of one kind of insulin into the vial of the other kind. It is advisable to draw up the smaller

Proper method of injecting insulin. The four drawings show the most important phases of insulin injection. *Upper left,* putting the syringe together. *Upper right,* pushing air into the insulin bottle. *Lower left,* drawing up of insulin. *Lower right,* injection of insulin.

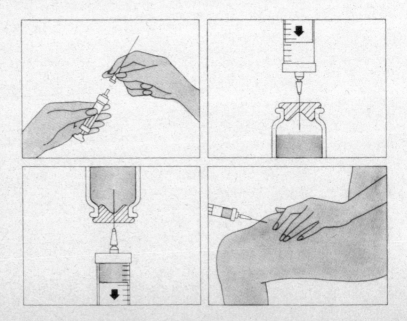

amount of insulin (regular insulin) first according to the procedure described above. Insert this partially filled syringe containing no air into the second insulin vial (air may be injected into it beforehand) and withdraw the necessary amount of insulin. Do not push any insulin back into the second bottle because the insulin in the second bottle would then be impure.

Injection techniques

proper injection technique

Firmly grasp a fold of tissue between the thumb and index finger of one hand, forming the widest possible fold. Grasp the syringe with the other hand like a pencil with the thumb, middle finger and index finger. If the needle is long (45 mm.) it should be inserted at an angle, and if short (11 mm.) insertion should be made perpendicularly to the fold of skin. The needle should be kept close to the skin before insertion thus making only a small pressure necessary to push the needle down to the desired depth.

After insertion, the thick fold of skin can be released, while a thin fold of skin should be held loosely between thumb and index finger. The plunger should be pushed down in a smooth movement, but not too quickly. The needle should be withdrawn in the same direction as inserted.

If the injection is performed properly, then the tip of the needle is located in subcutaneous fatty tissue. This is the case if light resistance is encountered while inserting the needle through the skin which is a little leather-like at the surface.

choosing the injection site

The choice of injection site is very important. Rotation of injection sites is important. If the injection sites are not rotated, then atrophy or painful scarring of the skin may occur. The best injection sites are the outside and front sides of the upper thigh, the outside of the upper arm, and the lower part of the abdominal skin and the buttocks.

mistakes when making an injection

The appearance of a small drop of blood should not cause concern unless it indicates that the injection was made into a blood vessel. To check, pull back the plunger a slight amount before injecting the insulin. If this is not the case, then part of the injected insulin may have entered the blood stream. Since this may cause hypoglycemia, the next meal should be consumed earlier.

If a white, usually painful, lump appears at the injection site,

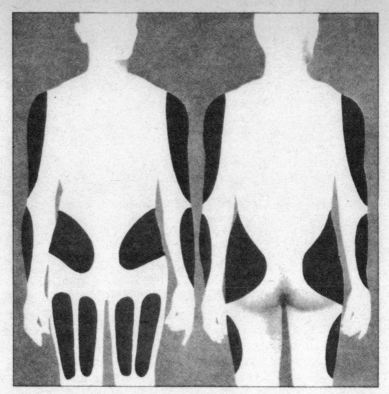

The most suitable sites for injection (left front side, right rear view). All sites which have subcutaneous fatty tissue are suitable (the dark areas in the drawing). The injection sites should be changed or rotated continuously in these areas.

then insulin was injected into the upper part of the skin instead of into subcutaneous fatty tissue. This is an error in injection technique which must be corrected.

allergy to insulin

In rare cases the skin becomes red at the injection site indicating an allergy to insulin, a defensive reaction of the body against the foreign substance. This reaction resembles a small inflammation. The so-called late reaction usually appears when the insulin is first used, and shows up at the injection site one or two weeks after the treatment with insulin is begun. The late reaction appears 24 to 48 hours after injection. Effective drugs are available to treat such allergic reactions. It is sometimes necessary to change the insulin type. Such reddening of skin at the injection site is not caused by an error in injection technique, uncleanliness or the use of alcohol to clean the syringe.

Finding the Balance among Insulin, Nutrition and Physical Activity

It is important to establish an exact schedule for the injections. The insulin injection should always be combined with meals and physical activity must be taken into consideration. It can happen that one does not anticipate engaging in physical activity. Hypoglycemia which may result from this situation can be prevented if measures are taken to adjust the metabolism. The following example shows which mistakes are likely to cause hypoglycemia.

improper balance

A student who oversleeps and is in a hurry to make it to school in time will probably not forget to inject insulin, since he knows this cannot be omitted. Being in a hurry, he does not eat his usual breakfast and eats a small amount hurriedly while taking the rest along. Since he is late, he runs to school. Hypoglycemia will probably occur since he has now lowered the blood sugar in two ways — first, with the insulin injection and secondly with the unusual physical activity that consumed sugar. At the same time, he did not eat enough carbohydrates at breakfast. The level of blood sugar decreases until hypoglycemia occurs. The student should have adhered to the strict procedure of properly timing the injection and consumption of the required amount of food instead of trying to be on time.

proper balance

Another example will show how the amount of insulin, intake of food, and physical activity must be balanced in cases of additional physical activity. This example involves an insulin dependent young diabetic who does not engage in physical activity during the week, but who likes sports on the weekend.

These examples show how important the timing and treatment adjustments can be for insulin dependent diabetics. Participation in different kinds of sports or increased physical activity during vacation may make it necessary to lower the insulin dosage prior to physical activity and increase the carbohydrate intake, both before and during the activity, according to the results of self-testing.

good timing between injection and meals

The diabetic must also balance the timing of the other measures of treatment in the daily routine. The insulin must always be injected before food is consumed. Prolonged action insulin, effective for a longer period of time, but slower reaching

77

Monday to Friday

Activity: *Office work, little physical activity*

Daily routine: On days without special physical activity the diabetic injects 28 units in the morning and 12 units in the evening of intermediate-acting insulin and consumes his six meals at the predetermined time. Regular self-testing will then show only small amounts of urinary sugar.

Principles governing treatment The methods of treatment are continued according to the same schedule with a careful balance between the insulin and food intake.

Saturday and Sunday

Activities *Sports on the weekend.*

Daily routine The first time the patient engages in soccer training on Saturday from 10 to 12 o'clock and participates in a game on Sunday at the same time, he ate only a little more in the morning. The resulting hypoglycemia forces him to interrupt the training and the game. On the following weekend, the patient reduces the first injection of insulin by 2 to 4 units (later maybe even 8 units) and eats more carbohydrates before the training. For example, an additional slice of bread might help him. The results of self-testing will show whether this change was sufficient to adjust to the increased physical activity.

Principles governing treatment Less insulin is injected before the sports event, for example 2 to 4 (up to 8) units. Increased intake of carbohydrates before sports (an extra slice of bread) make it possible for the diabetic to participate in sports.

its peak, must be injected 30 minutes prior to breakfast or dinner. Short or intermediate acting insulin must be injected about 15 minutes before the meals.

Insulin-Induced Hypoglycemia

The most frequent side effect of the insulin dependent diabetic is hypoglycemia in the daily routine. This is not a true side effect, but a sign of the effectiveness of insulin. Hypoglycemia should not be seen as an isolated effect requiring an immediate change in the insulin dose. This condition is always the consequence of an inadequate balance between nutrition, physical activity and insulin treatment. Hypoglycemia may be caused by improper nutrition or unexpected physical activity.

most com-
mon causes
of hypo-
glycemia

All insulin dependent diabetics must be able to recognize the symptoms of hypoglycemia in order to take correct measures against it. Two kinds of symptoms are differentiated. Some symptoms are the result of autonomic nervous system stim-

Symptoms of hypoglycemia

Resulting from stimulation of autonomic nervous system:

restlessness	trembling
fear	palpitations
sweating	sudden craving for food
pallor	sensations of hot and cold

Resulting from glucose deficiency of brain cells:

headaches	peculiar behavior
difficulty in concentration	(aggressive, euphoric)
difficulty in remembering	absent-mindedness
double vision	sleepiness
dizziness	confusion
difficulty in walking	speech disturbances
straight	unconsciousness
tingling around the mouth	convulsions

79

ulation, whereas other complaints are the result of sudden glucose deficiency in brain cells. Severe symptoms appear only rarely and can be prevented or treated in time just as less severe complications can. Each diabetic should be aware of his individual reaction in hypoglycemia. There is no list of symptoms which can be applied to all because the reaction varies in intensity and speed from one diabetic to the next.

Hypoglycemia is probably most frequently the result of omitting a usual and necessary meal, or of consuming it late or incompletely. An example of this case is the diabetic student who overslept and is in such a hurry that he neglects the proper balance between diet and insulin. Often the morning snack is omitted, causing hypoglycemia before lunch. Instead of reducing the amount of insulin injected in the morning, care should be taken to adhere to the meal schedule. Sometimes a third snack in the morning is necessary to control the metabolism, as for example in diabetic children with long school hours.

We certainly hope you will not develop hypoglycemia, but an experience of a mild hypoglycemic state may help you understand and achieve better control of your metabolism. The symptoms need not be severe, because only the first few signals are necessary for recognition and determination of measures to be taken. The use of the term "shock" does not have the same meaning in this context as for someone experiencing severe hypoglycemia. The term "shock" refers only to hypoglycemia itself.

Light cases of hypoglycemia need not always be treated. When there is a sugar deficiency, the liver excretes its reserve sugar into the blood, thus causing a temporary improvement. The diabetic should nevertheless undertake some corrective measure when the first symptoms appear in order to avoid further lowering of the blood sugar.

Pure sugar serves this purpose well. In such an extreme situation, a lump of sugar, candy or very sweet drinks are not only permitted but necessary. They are a simple measure of treatment because they are quickly absorbed from the stomach and small intestine. In the case of light shock, fruit juice, fruit, bread or immediate consumption of the next meal may be sufficient measures of treatment. Foods rich in carbohydrates with additional fats are not suitable, because they require more time to be absorbed (for example, sandwiches, cake or chocolate.).

carry sugar with you

Diabetics who may develop hypoglycemia, and insulin dependent diabetics in particular, must always carry sugar in a suitable form with them. Although the diabetic should not consume pure sugar every day, he must keep some available for hypoglycemia. The diabetic should think of the places he visits during the day and keep a provision of sugar at the places most frequently used. He may wish to keep sugar in his apartment (also near the bed for the night), at his place of work, and also in a wallet (or pocketbook), jacket pocket, and, certainly, in the car.

apple or bread for an emergency

At the onset of hypoglycemia, the patient should consume a glass of apple juice, three or four lumps of sugar, or one to two pieces of toast. If this has no effect after five minutes, then the patient should consume another small quantity of sugar. In this process, the patient will learn how much sugar to take in overcoming his hypoglycemia. If the quantity is too large, then the blood sugar level will be elevated. Concentrated sugar should be consumed only in the case of acute or severe hypoglycemia, but not in impending or light cases. An experienced diabetic knows that in the case of light hypoglycemia, an apple or slice of bread may be more suitable because he can avoid a strong elevation of blood sugar level and at the same time treat his hypoglycemia.

relatives should be informed

Relatives and friends of the diabetic should be informed about the disease and also about hypoglycemia. They should know the symptoms and what must be done in an extreme case of unconsciousness. Instructions concerning hypoglycemia should be noted in the identification card of the diabetic so that others unfamiliar with the disease could help. It is important to notify the physician when hypoglycemia has occurred. Under no conditions should an unconscious patient be force-fed with sweet liquids. If glucagon is available, then this hormone which elevates blood sugar can be injected in fatty tissue or muscle. The diabetic must consume carbohydrates immediately after awakening to build up the sugar reserves in the body again.

Side Effects of Insulin

One of the side effects of insulin treatment is hypersensitivity of the skin, indicating the body's incompatibility with the insulin. The symptoms of this allergy are itching, redness and swelling at and around the injection site. Only the physician can decide whether this is temporary and will disappear after two or three weeks, or whether the type of insulin must be changed.

Some diabetics may react to insulin injections over a long period of time with atrophy. Although these disturbances are harmless, they can be bothersome for cosmetic reasons. Atrophy can be avoided by regular rotation of the injection site.

Finally, visual disorders with far-sightedness occur relatively frequently when insulin treatment is begun. They are caused by the re-adaption of the lenses of the eyeball to normal blood sugar values after having first adjusted to higher blood sugar concentrations. Although this problem with far-sightedness is temporary and usually disappears after two to four weeks, it could mean that the diabetic will be restricted in his permission to drive. Since these complaints disappear after a short period, it is not necessary to have a pair of glasses prescribed.

9. Physical Activity and Sports

Physical activity and exercise are as important as diet and medication. It is necessary to keep a balance between these three treatment modalities.

The diabetic must be encouraged to engage in vigorous physical activity. The best influence on metabolism occurs when the patient exercises to the point of perspiring. The positive effect of this exercise is to increase the uptake of glucose by the muscles without requiring additional insulin. It can be said in an oversimplification that exercise has the effect of an additional injection of insulin. But exercise can have this positive effect only if the metabolism is balanced. If it is out of control, then exercise may have a negative influence. In this case exercise would worsen the metabolic condition.

All diabetics whose metabolism is balanced can be physically active. However, not all kinds of sports are suited to the diabetic. When choosing a particular type of exercise, the patient should consider the following requirements:

proper choice of sports

the right amount of exercise

- The type of sport must be suited to his physical condition at the moment. Overexertion can have a negative influence on the general well-being
- An exercise should be chosen which requires endurance rather than a temporary peak of performance in which energy is consumed all at once.
- It should be possible to perform the chosen exercise without elaborate equipment.

Among the many forms of exercise which fulfill these requirements are the following: floor exercises, cross country running or walking, gymnastics, sports involving teams (handball, soccer, volleyball, hockey, ping-pong), medium distance races, bicycling, sledding, roller skating, rowing, tennis, skating, swimming, cross country and downhill skiing.

Even older diabetics who did not engage in sports earlier can participate in physical activity which fulfills the previous requirements. They will quickly learn to strike a balance between physical activity and control of blood sugar level. There are many forms of exercise which do not entail a health hazard. The following forms are recommended:

Jogging: alternating periods of jogging and walking allow the patient to increase endurance in an excellent manner. Prerequisites are healthy feet and legs and joints, and no back problems.

Bicycling: recommended for those who are not well-trained. Almost anyone can learn bicycling since it does not require great physical ability. It is not likely that the untrained person will overexert himself, because only one part of the musculature is used and these muscles will grow tired before the heart does.

The static burden on the joints is minimal, although the knee joints must be in good functioning condition.

Swimming: this is fun and healthy because all major muscles are employed in a uniform way. Swimming pools can be found almost everwhere and mechanical overburdening of the joints is not possible. (This is particularly important for the obese). The buoyancy of the water lifts the body.

Hiking: this is not the same as a leisurely walk. It is good exercise only if a distance of 3 to 5 miles (5 to 8 kilometers) with both uphill and downhill portions is covered in an hour. Good shoes and clothes according to weather conditions should be worn. In the winter, hiking can be performed as cross country skiing.

professional sports possible

These recommendations are intended above all for the older diabetic. A young diabetic not suffering from any other organic disease may choose other forms of sport. The diabetic should always take care to adjust physical activity to the individual blood sugar needs. Young diabetics sometimes ask whether they can engage in professional sports. Professional tennis players who participated in the Davis Cup Finals are good examples of successful diabetic athletes. Recently a German hockey player who participated in the Olympic games and world championship games reported that his diabetes did not interfere with physical activity. These examples show that young insulin-dependent diabetics do not necessarily run the risk of a health hazard when engaged in tennis or hockey even if periods of stress cannot be anticipated. It is possible to engage in professional sports if training is well planned, if appropriate measures are taken before training (less insulin, more carbohydrates), and if proper measures are taken when the first signs of hypoglycemia appear.

Most diabetics are probably not interested in professional sports. These may still enjoy exercise and favorably influence their metabolism without forcing themselves and without the desire to compete. We recommend that all diabetics who are physically capable of exercise do participate in physical activity. Diabetic children should be allowed to participate in sports in school and in clubs if they desire to do so. There is no reason to forbid a diabetic child from engaging in sports if he is capable of recognizing the first signs of hypoglycemia and of taking the necessary measures for treatment.

10. Regular Checkups

We have already described the goals of good treatment of diabetes:

Goals of good diabetes treatment

Good treatment should:
- avoid worsening the diabetes
- prevent acute dangers from occurring
- help prevent or delay vascular damage

Good treatment allows the patient to obtain:
- physical and emotional well-being
- normal productive capacity
- unimpeded participation in family, professional and social life
- favorable life-expectancy

you can also attain these goals

These goals can be attained only if the effectiveness of treatment is regularly controlled in examinations.

An attempt must be made daily to control the blood sugar level. Obviously, self-testing of metabolism must be added to the results of the medical examination to meet this challenge. Such combined testing will make it possible for the patient to be informed about his present situation and to adjust methods of treatment to individual needs.

Medical Examinations

Since the absence of urinary sugar, and the values for blood sugar, body weight, and blood lipids should be as close to normal as possible to control diabetes, the physician will weigh the patient and test the concentration of sugar in the blood and urine each time the patient appears for consultation. The blood lipids should be tested at least twice a year.

blood tests

The metabolic condition and methods of treatment used determine the frequency with which the physician performs these tests. If the medical examination shows poor metabolic condition, then the physican will ask the patient to return within a short period of time. If, however, the condition is favorable, then fewer examinations will be necessary. Those insulin-dependent diabetics whose blood sugar values fluctuate greatly, must be seen more regularly than those treated with diet alone or with oral hypoglycemic agents and whose metabolic condition tends to remain in balance.

Usually, medical examinations are performed once every four weeks on insulin-dependent diabetics. A patient who is treated with diet alone or in combination with oral hypoglycemic agents should be examined every eight weeks.

Blood sugar is tested either when the diabetic is fasting, or after one hour following a meal. The patient should always bring a quantitative urine sample, which means that he should collect urine from a 24 hour period and then bring a sample for the medical consultation.

quantitative urine test

The urine sample allows the physician to draw conclusions concerning the blood sugar values during the 24 hour collection period. For example, if the urine does not indicate any sugar, then one can assume the blood sugar was not higher than 180 mg/100 ml during this time. Why? Knowledge about the renal threshold provides part of the answer. Sugar is excreted in urine only if the blood sugar rises above 180 mg/100 ml. The answer to the frequent question "What is worse, blood sugar or urinary sugar?" is now obvious. One value is not worse than another, because both are closely linked and provide information about the course of blood sugar values.

Another integral part of the regular medical examination is the physical examination, taking of the blood pressure (which must be performed more frequently if elevated), x-ray of the lung, and the EKG. Diabetics who suffer from no other diseases may omit some of these yearly medical examinations. Certain conditions may make it necessary to perform additional tests, such as a particular examination of the urine when a bladder inflammation or renal problems are suspected. All diabetics should have a yearly eye examination performed to determine whether any vessels have been damaged in the retina. If such damage has occurred then examination should be repeated frequently. Treatment must begin at the proper time. It is possible to treat vessel damage of the retina by laser beams today. The painless technique of laser coagulation is used to form a scar over these

eye examination

diseased parts of the retina to prevent further damage to the vessels.

Self-Testing of Urinary and Blood Sugar

The physician must advise and instruct the diabetic how to plan, calculate and maintain proper nutrition. The diabetic must take his medicine and inject insulin himself. The diabetic must be able to interpret the results of his metabolism himself.

The purpose of self-testing and of medical examination is an early recognition of deterioration in the condition, allowing the diabetic to make necessary adjustments in his treatment. If the patient informs his physician of the changes he observes, then the physican will be able to take corrective measures. The diabetic can also learn to adjust his own treatment measures within certain limits.

Information about weight and the results of urinary sugar tests are the basic elements of regular self-testing. Occasionally it may also be necessary to test the acetone in the urine. Generally speaking, the patient will not have to perform blood sugar tests because these are suited more to recognition of extreme situations such as very high or very low blood sugar levels.

treatment must be readjusted

methods of self-testing

Methods for self-testing of metabolism

- Body weight:
  daily weight control

- Urinary sugar:
  Clinitest (Five drop is standard, and two drop), Clinistix, Diastix, Tes-tape, Multi-stix, Acetest, Ketostix, Combistix, Keto diastix, **Chemstrip G,** Benedict's solution

- Acetone in the urine:
  Acetest, **Ketostix,** Keto-diastix, "Acetone Test" powder (Denver Chemical Manuf. Co.)

- Blood sugar:
  Dextrostix, **Chemstrip bG**

(The methods in heavy type are the ones recommended)

The urinary sugar test

All diabetics must perform the urinary sugar test as a part of the self-testing program. The physician will determine which test should be used.

strip tests

There are two basic types of urinary tests: test strips are briefly dipped into the urine, whereas test tablets require that a certain amount of urine (and perhaps a specific number of drops of water as well) be placed on the tablet. Contact with the urine initiates a chemical reaction in the testing material. If the urine contains sugar, then the strip is discolored within 60 seconds. A scale is provided to measure this discoloration so that the sugar concentration can be estimated.

The more precise the method employed, the clearer is the result. Experience has shown that the Chemstrip G is the most accurate method for determination of urinary sugar content even in the presence of vitamin C intake. In addition, two methods of Clinitest are available: the five-drop method indicates blood sugar concentrations up to 2% (that is, 2 grams per 100 cc. urine), and the two-drop method permitting identification of 3% and 5% urinary sugar levels (3 and 5 grams per 100 cc. urine). The package insert explains how these methods are employed. If the result of the five-drop method indicates a concentration above 2%, then a test with the two-drop method should be performed to estimate the higher concentration. The only difference in the use of the two methods is the number of drops. There is also a different color chart.

keep a record

The diabetic should record his results. Comparison of these results will indicate the time of day when excess urinary sugar is excreted. Appropriate changes can then be made in the treatment. These results may be discussed with the physician during the next medical consultation.

Clinitest, color chart and reading

It does not matter whether the results are noted as numbers on a prepared chart, in a booklet supplied by the manufacturer, or noted as colors. Notation of colors may be suited for children who can recognize elevated sugar values more easily in the form of colors than numbers.

Dip the paper strip into the urine for one second, tap the strip against the edge of the container to remove excess urine and wait one minute before comparing the test area to the color chart. The chart shows increments of +1, +2, +3, +4 which indicate

.1%, .5%, 1%, and 2% respectively of sugar concentration.

Some of the other tests permit only a determination of whether or not sugar is present. If the urine contains sugar, the test strip is discolored to varying degrees, but these shadings cannot be used to measure the exact amount present. If the urine contains no sugar, then no discoloration occurs.

Acetone test

Testing the urine for acetone is advisable when the sugar concentration is great. It is sufficient to simply test for the presence of acetone. Its presence is an important indication of an impending or already established serious metabolic disorder.

For the examination the acetest tablet is placed on a clean piece of white paper or white paper towel. A drop of urine is placed on the tablet. If acetone is present, the tablet turns lavender or light purple. Ketostix also turns lavender or purple when the strip test is dipped into urine containing acetone.

Self-testing of the blood sugar

It is usually unnecessary to test the blood sugar since it does not add more precise information to the urinary test results. The self-testing of blood sugar is recommended for diabetic patients who have a tendency to develop hypoglycemia, as is often the case in diabetic children.

Quick methods for self-determination of blood sugar values include the Chemstrip bG. First the tip of the finger is cleaned with an alcohol swab. Then a small sharp needle is used to puncture the skin. The first drop of blood which appears is placed on the test zone of the paper strip. The entire test zone must be covered with blood. If the Chemstrip bG is used, then the test zone is wiped three times, but does not need to be washed with water. The color of the test zone is compared to the color chart to estimate the concentration of sugar in the blood.

Adjusting Treatment to Results of Self-Testing

The diabetic who is treated with diet and oral hypoglycemic agents has gained control over the blood sugar level only if the highest blood sugar value during the day does not exceed the renal threshold, a value of 160-180 mg/100 ml. In this case, the diabetic is not excreting sugar into the urine. For this purpose, the self-testing with test strips is sufficient in the diabetic treated with diet and oral hypoglycemic agents. If sugar is found in the urine, he obviously has not gained control.

several urine samples

The diabetic should perform a quantitative test, which means that he should collect urine for 24 hours or from the previous day and night. He should then test a sample taken from the total amount of urine to determine whether sugar was present. Or the physician may want to perform the quantitative test in his lab.

For many diabetic patients, such a quantitative test is not only unnecessary, but superfluous. The insulin-dependent diabetic should instead perform four urinary tests in the course of the day using the Chemstrip G. The following times are recommended for testing: fasting in the morning, before lunch, before dinner, and before retiring to sleep. If the fasting urinary test in the morning indicates the presence of sugar in the urine, then this means that blood sugar exceeded the renal threshold during the night. In this case, the dose of insulin taken in the evening was insufficient and must be readjusted.

The test taken before lunch indicates whether the blood sugar exceeded the renal threshold during the morning and whether the insulin injected in the morning was insufficient. If urinary sugar was excreted before dinner, then the blood sugar in the afternoon exceeded the renal threshold, demonstrating that the insulin injected in the morning was insufficient for the afternoon.

The test performed before retiring to sleep in the evening indicates whether the evening dose of insulin was sufficient for the amount of carbohydrates consumed at the dinner.

half-hour urine test

More accurate results can be gained if the urine is examined half an hour after the first urination. For this test the urine is voided and then disposed of. After half an hour has passed, the diabetic drinks a glass of water or tea to stimulate urination and repeats the testing of the urine. This method permits the gathering of a sample of urine produced during the last 30 minutes. If sugar is present in this urine, then the blood sugar level exceeded renal threshold in the last 30 minutes, indicating that it is above the level 160-180 mg/100 ml within that time period. This method yields precise information about the blood sugar values of the preceding half hour.

This half hour test of the urine can also be performed at other times during the day. It should be employed when a quick decision must be reached about the additional amount of insulin needed in the case of metabolic disorders resulting, for example, from a serious sickness accompanied by fever or loss of appetite.

11. What the Diabetic Should Also Know

This detailed discussion of diabetes treatment and the ways in which the physician determines what the patient has to do should clarify the goal of this treatment method: the diabetic should adjust his daily routine to the requirements imposed on him by diabetes so that he may lead a healthy and happy life.

the diabetic's conditional health

A diabetologist, Professor Katsch, once formulated the phrase "conditional health" of the diabetic, which all diabetics can achieve if they control their blood sugar level.

In the following, we shall present a few of the diabetic's problems. Some of these are purely medical problems and others are everyday situations to which diabetics must react differently than a normal person.

Personal Hygiene As a Preventive Measure

especially important for the diabetic

Surely good personal hygiene ought to be practiced by everyone, but the diabetic must be particularly aware of this because he is more susceptible to general infections, inflammatory diseases of the skin and dental problems. The diabetic should therefore take a shower or bath once a day. He should wash his hands after each meal, after using the lavatory, and after working.

91

The feet of the diabetic are exposed to particularly dangerous situations when there are circulatory problems or nervous disorders, particularly after injury or infection. Gangrene is a possible threat. Good foot care is essential.

Rules of foot care for the diabetic
- Wash feet daily (never use very hot water) using mild soap and rinsing the feet well. After drying the feet and the area between the toes thoroughly, examine all blisters, wounds, abrasions or skin discolorations carefully.
- Skin care: Rub salve on dry and chapped skin twice a day. Use regular powder for perspiration. Apply special salve to callouses. Callouses are pressure points and this pressure must be relieved.
- It is best to cut or file nails shortly after a footbath, taking care *not to cut them too closely.* Avoid injuring the cuticles.
- Wear a fresh pair of socks every day and, if possible, a pair made of cotton, yarn or terrycloth; tight elastic should be avoided.
- Always wear shoes to avoid injury to the feet. Take care to choose the correct size and well-fitting shoes, and wear shoes or boots made of rubber only for sports and bad weather. Do not walk barefoot.
- Do gymnastic exercises to strengthen the muscles of the foot.
- If problems are encountered with foot care, a podiatrist should be seen immediately. If the feet change or complications appear, the physician must be consulted.

rules for dental care

Proper dental care is also particularly important for the diabetic patient. Diabetics suffer not only more frequently from cavities than healthy people, but also from diseased gums, roots and periodontal membrane, as well as the jaw and facial bones.

Formation of plaque following meals should be prevented by brushing teeth. For this reason, it is important to brush the teeth for three minutes after each meal. Time yourself with a watch to make sure that actual brushing time is three minutes. At the very least, the teeth should be brushed after breakfast and dinner.

The most suitable toothbrushes are those made from synthetic materials which have rounded tips. If the proper brushing technique is used, then the area between teeth is also reached.

Electric toothbrushes may also be employed. Another method which may be used in conjunction with brushing (but should not replace the toothbrush) is a jet of water to clean out food particles which may remain in areas reached only with great difficulty by a toothbrush.

Any brand of toothpaste is acceptable. The fluoride contained in toothpaste is important for the maintenance of the teeth.

Concomitant Illness

what about
your blood
pressure?

Many diabetics have an elevated blood pressure, insufficient cardiac output or blood supply from the heart, or their blood lipids may be elevated. Older diabetics in particular may suffer from other diseases such as gout (elevation of uric acid) and inflammation of the urinary tract. These diseases are usually chronic and they must be subjected to constant control and drug therapy.

As a result, older diabetics in particular must often take other drugs in addition to the oral hypoglycemic agents. It is no wonder that many diabetics sometimes forget to take a pill or consciously neglect to take the recommended pills because there are so many to take. Although the patient may be aware of the harmful effect this can have on the body, he may still neglect to take the pills because no immediate pain results. High blood pressure, elevated lipid values, and elevated uric acid values in the blood do not cause symptoms for many years and harmful consequences become noticeable only after asymptomatic decades.

Perhaps you also belong to this group of diabetics who must take a number of pills by doctor's orders and wish that there were not so many. This wish is easy to fulfill if you are overweight, like the vast majority of adult diabetics: make an honest attempt to lose weight. Weight reduction lowers the blood pressure and normalizes the blood lipids, in addition to relieving the strain on the heart. Rather than beginning by neglecting the pills, a patient should begin by reducing weight. The physician will then determine how many pills must still be taken.

If Unable to Eat

The sudden onset of an illness requires that the measures of

93

treatment be modified immediately to suit this new situation. Such readjustment will test the patient's knowledge and ensure proper self-testing on healthy days.

fever, nausea, vomiting

In the case of acute illness the patient is no longer capable or has no desire to consume his usual meals, as for example when an infection causes high fever; when an upset stomach or intestinal disorder causes nausea or vomiting; when there is some other cause for loss of appetite. The patient must then decide how to best continue his treatment. Should an insulin-dependent diabetic decide not to inject insulin because he cannot eat anything that day, then he risks a severe metabolic disorder and coma.

From time to time it is necessary to reduce the amount of insulin or the number of pills when the patient cannot eat at all or cannot eat his normal amount. Which guidelines must then be followed? The amount of insulin or the number of tablets is determined by the results of repeated urinary sugar tests. If these tests indicate the presence of urinary sugar or acetone in the urine, then the patient should inject the usual amount of insulin despite the fact that he can hardly eat due to nausea or vomiting. The patient should repeat these tests each time he urinates. It is absolutely essential that the physician be informed.

first aid until physician arrives

If the patient must undertake some form of treatment himself because he cannot reach the physician or a hospital, then he should use the results of the urinary sugar and acetone tests as guidelines for the following hours. If the tests continue to show positive results 3 or 4 hours after the usual injection, then the patient should inject an additional 4 to 6 units of short-acting insulin. A bottle of such rapid acting insulin must be kept for such emergencies, even if the patient normally injects a different kind of insulin. If this additional injection of insulin does not change the strong positive readings of the urinary sugar and acetone tests after 3 or 4 hours, then the same amount of insulin should be injected again. As soon as test results indicate a slight improvement, no more short-acting insulin should be injected, since this injection could cause hypoglycemia. It would be best to drink small amounts of liquids — tea or water — and to try to eat porridge or oatmeal. The patient should not forget to inject his usual dose of insulin once the threat has passed.

The following guidelines have been established for the diabetic

94

who must undertake his own treatment. The Swiss diabetologist, Dr. Constam, has called these the "zero to eight" rules. If the urinary sugar does not decrease, then the amounts of insulin should be adjusted to the results of the Clinitest 5-drop method:
Clinitest blue (= negative urinary sugar): 0 units of short-acting insulin.
Clinitest green (= ¼ to ¾% urinary sugar or trace amounts to 2+): 2 units of short-acting insulin.
Clinitest brown (= 1% urinary sugar or 3+): 4 units of short-acting insulin.
Clinitest orange (= 2% urinary sugar or more or 4+): 8 units of short-acting insulin.

The patient should ask his physician whether these recommended doses are suited to his individual case. These guidelines are valid for diabetics who require a usual daily dose of 40 units, but must be readjusted for those requiring different amounts of insulin.

bringing un-usual situa-tions under control

Of course, these guidelines should be followed in all cases where patients do not consume the usual meal. They may be followed in other extreme situations as, for example, on long flights with irregular food intake and complete inactivity. The unique case of an insulin dependent diabetic forced to spend several days on a hijacked plane, who was allowed to eat only from time to time and who was dependent on unfamiliar insulin, demonstrates the effectiveness of such measures. This diabetic proved how important it is for the patient to readjust his insulin dose according to the results of the urinary sugar test in this extreme situation. Other diabetics should be able to handle a temporary acute illness in everyday life equally well.

Problem Medications

Sometimes medications prescribed for other illnesses influence the blood sugar values and thus the metabolism of the diabetic. Certain medication increases the blood sugar making it necessary for the diabetic to readjust his dose of insulin. Tonics and cough syrups may contain pure sugar and should therefore be avoided by the diabetic.

caution advised for cough syrup

Some drugs lower the blood sugar by increasing the effect of sulfonylurea pills. Since the risk of hypoglycemia is then

95

increased, the diabetic should take preventive measures by readjusting his nutrition.

The diabetic must know which drugs can affect the results of his urinary sugar and acetone tests.

Medication which can interfere with metabolism and urinary sugar tests

Worsening of metabolic conditions
 Epinephrine
 Corticosteroids
 Oral contraceptives
 Diuretics
 Nicotinic acid
 Medications containing sugar

Lower blood sugar
 anticoagulants (dicumarol)
 drugs for rheumatism (butazolidin)
 sulfonylureas
 pain killers and drugs against fevers containing salicylates

Interferes with urinary sugar testing
(depends on method used)
 Vitamin C
 Pyrazolone
 Salicylates
 Tetracyclines
 Penicillin
 Isonicotinic acid
 Para-aminosalicylic acid

The Diabetic in the Hospital

surgery — no higher risk

It may become necessary for the diabetic to be admitted to the hospital for treatment of another disease; for example, he may need surgery. If the blood sugar level is under control, then surgery does not cause any threat. The patient who is worried that his diabetes may cause problems can be reassured that this is not the case. It appears that a diabetic whose blood sugar is under control runs no higher risk during surgery than a non-diabetic patient.

The patient can prepare himself for an anticipated stay in the hospital, whether for surgery or treatment of another disease. He should take pertinent information about his treatment to the hospital with him, including the medicine he is taking, his diet plan, his diabetes identification card, the results of his metabolic tests, details pertaining to his diabetes and its course, as well as earlier measures of treatment or test results from other examinations (for example, eye examinations, EKG, blood pressure values or earlier medical records.). This information may make it possible to hasten treatment and shorten the stay in the hospital.

Relationships and Sexuality

Learning to live with diabetes involves participation of the spouse in mastering the problems and tasks of diabetes. How can one's partner help? He or she must not only be ready to help, but must also be well-informed in order to be of assistance. Problems arise in three general areas: the actual treatment of diabetes, the normalization of everyday life, and in diabetic men in particular, sexuality.

You have probably been aware of the vital role of your spouse in treating your diabetes for a long time already. You have probably appreciated this help in planning meals, in injecting insulin or in the treatment of a hypoglycemic episode.

It is more difficult to help when the diabetic has problems in his professional and social life. The spouse of the diabetic will not be able to step in, for example, if the diabetic has problems at his job, is not promoted, if he has problems with his driver's license or when he is regarded as a second-rate person in his circle of friends.

The relationship may nonetheless be satisfying if the partners cooperate in mastering the problem, learning from these attempts and demonstrating to those around them that the diabetic is not truly sick, but can lead a completely normal and productive life.

Sexuality may become a particular problem for diabetic men. We know from many conversations that he will hesitate to speak about this problem with a physician (or with his spouse) and that he will appreciate it if the physician mentions this topic.

Almost half of all diabetic men notice some degree of

97

decreased sexual ability, which may manifest itself in different forms. While some may experience difficulty with erection, but no decrease in sexual desire, others observe decreased interest. Disturbances in sexual performance may lead to impotence and problems with sexual desire are disturbances of libido.

Metabolic disorders or a long-term poor metabolic condition may cause acute disturbance of potency. Once the metabolic condition is normalized, the disturbances in potency will soon disappear.

Treatment of chronic sexual problems not accompanied by poor metabolism is much more difficult. Since there usually is not any hormonal imbalance, there is no reason to engage in any hormonal treatment. A disorder of the nervous function in the pelvic area is often found in diabetics, but unfortunately no general treatment has been discovered for this problem. For this reason, treatment in the form of constant control of the metabolism becomes all the more important.

other causes of impotence

Disturbance of potency in diabetics may also be caused by other factors, for instance certain drugs which have such side effects, or the causes may be emotional rather than physical in nature. The patient should not hesitate to consult the physician and ask for help.

talk with your partner

These difficulties should also be discussed with the spouse. The diabetic should tell his spouse about his anxiety. It is, of course, self-evident and acknowledged as true by all that sexuality is a fundamental part of our lives and must be maintained as such. Sex is a way of attaining personal self-fulfillment and a unique form of happiness with one's spouse for most persons, whether healthy or sick, old or young. The couple should cooperate to solve problems which may arise.

Family Planning

Genetic predisposiion to develop diabetes is passed from one generation to the next. Geneticists still do not know exactly how the genetic material is transmitted. If a diabetic asks what the chances are that his child may have diabetes, we can only give him the unsatisfactory statistical answer of the geneticist.

risk for your fetus?

The risk of developing diabetes during one's lifetime (not only to inherit the predisposition) is about 10% if one parent is

98

diabetic, but the other is not. There is only a 1 to 2% chance that a person in this situation will become insulin dependent before age 40. If the other parent is not diabetic, but carries genes for diabetes, then there is a 50% chance that the child will also develop diabetes.

The greatest risk of developing diabetes is about 60% in children both of whose parents are diabetic. These parents should not have children for this reason. Patients who cannot have children for medical reasons or who decide against it must choose a reliable method of contraception. Much information and medical advice is available on the methods which a woman or man may employ.

Planned Pregnancy

Prior to the discovery of insulin, pregnancy was rare in diabetic women and almost always entailed the mother's death. Today, however, it is the child who is the focal point of discussion concerning pregnancy and diabetes. The incidence of miscarriages and fatal consequences are more frequent in children of diabetics than in children of healthy women. Children of diabetic women whose blood sugar was uncontrolled before and during the pregnancy are at high risk. The better the control of metabolism and the smaller the number of complications which arise, the lower the risk of serious problems, which may be no more than for normal women.

precautionary
measures
during
pregnancy

A diabetic woman who decides to have a child should plan the pregnancy far in advance. An essential part of this planning is the control of blood sugar level. The medical examination which must be performed before the pregnancy may indicate an elevated risk if there are changes in the blood vessels or kidney disease.

Planning also includes the readiness to undergo more medical examinations and self-tests than were necessary before the pregnancy. If diabetes can be controlled during pregnancy, then the child's risk is diminished considerably. Specialized medical consultation is important during the last weeks of pregnancy and at the time of birth. Centers in which experienced teams of obstetricians, pediatricians and diabetologists can cooperate offer the best treatment.

99

What the pregnant diabetic woman must know

- Good diabetes control is necessary in order to prevent endangering the fetus.
- The incidence of hypoglycemia is higher in the first trimester of pregnancy but the fetus is not endangered. Insulin requirements eventually decrease.
- After this period the insulin requirement usually increases and the dose must be increased from two injections per day to three.
- The renal threshold decreases during the third trimester of pregnancy and urinary sugar may appear even though the blood sugar values are normal. For this reason, only the blood sugar results may be used as guides.
- Weight gain during pregnancy should be limited to 22 to 24 pounds (10 to 11 kilograms). A high level of urinary sugar and acetone in the urine indicates that the metabolism is no longer under control. Since the fetus is acutely endangered the physician must be consulted immediately.
- During pregnancy blood pressure and body weight must be measured once a week if possible. A rise in blood pressure can be the first indication of a kidney disturbance. The physician must be consulted.
- The eyes should be checked once a month if possible in order to permit early recognition of changes in the retina and immediate treatment with laser beams (harmless even during pregnancy).
- The woman should deliver her child in a hospital where experienced physicians (internist, obstetrician, pediatrician) cooperate in a team. Since diabetic women usually deliver sooner than women with a normal metabolism, they must be admitted to the hospital earlier.
- Since the child of a diabetic woman is endangerd, the hospital must be equipped with an intensive care unit for premature infants.
- Shortly after the delivery, the increased insulin requirement temporarily drops to a very low level and then rises back to the amount required before pregnancy.

The Diabetic at Work

learning to
live with
diabetes

The capacity and readiness of a person to perform well professionally largely determines his standing in society. This aspect of our society may cause the diabetic family professional or social problems.

The diabetic is sometimes discriminated against when he is employed because diabetes is considered to be a serious illness which lowers his job performance and which imposes a burden on his employer. This judgment is not justified. Extensive studies have shown that work absenteeism is no higher and sometimes even lower among diabetics than among healthy persons.

Diabetics can hold almost any job and can be as productive as healthy persons. However, diabetes may cause certain problems when the diabetic exercises his profession. A diabetic whose illness was diagnosed before he began to work and who was able to choose his work site to match the special needs of his problem can best solve these difficulties. Some jobs are not suited or less suitable for the diabetic. Unsuitable jobs include those offering no opportunity to follow a diet and to control the metabolism regularly; moreover, jobs which require irregular hours of work are also not suited for the diabetic. Jobs in which the diabetic poses a risk to the safety of others and himself by the onset of hypoglycemia, for example, are also not suitable.

suitable —
unsuitable
jobs

Aside from these exceptions, the diabetic can choose from a wide range of other professions which allow him to control the metabolism without great difficulty. The most suitable jobs are those which involve working a regular number of hours, a well-balanced measure of physical activity, and the possibility to follow the meal plan and perform self-testing of the metabolism.

Problems sometimes arise when the diabetic desires to work in civil service. If he meets the requirements for the job and can perform his treatment measures at the work site, then his acceptance for the job is not a medical problem. In the United States, most Civil Service jobs are open to diabetics because the U.S. Civil Service Commission has taken a very progressive attitude toward diabetics. The regulations established by the U.S. Civil Service Commission state that "all diabetics who have achieved reasonable control over the condition are eligible for federal employment with proper placement to be based on the

101

Unsuitable jobs for diabetics

Jobs a diabetic may not hold because there is a risk to general safety	Locomotive engineers, pilots, captains, crane drivers, drivers for public transportation, driving large trucks, gateman for trains
Jobs which endanger the safety of the diabetic himself	Roofer, chimney sweep, mason, working with high voltage wires, installation of telephone posts, fire fighter, working with blast furnaces, or as a miner
Jobs not suitable because of difficulties following the diet	Innkeeper, cook, confectioner, baker, waiter, brewer, grocer
Jobs with irregular hours	Businessman, artist, shift worker

Recommended jobs for diabetics

Highly recommended jobs	Physician, dentist, pharmacist, nurse, physical therapist, technical assistant, physician's assistant, laboratory assistant, dietician
Recommended jobs	Employees and officials in hospitals, research institutes, public health departments; jobs in teaching and in churches
Jobs with sufficient prerequisites	Technical jobs such as mechanic, technician, working with low voltage electrical current, technical drawing, craftsmen such as gardener or locksmith, commercial artist

severity of the diabetes and the medication required for control."

If an older person who has specialized in working as a truck or bus driver, for example, suddenly develops diabetes, then he must find a new job. Persons who develop complications from long-term diabetes may also have to change their jobs, such as the clock-maker who is suddenly plagued by blurred vision. The diabetic should then be re-trained for a new job. Some diabetics prefer not to allow anyone in their professional environment to know their condition. These diabetics fear discrimination and feel that terms such as "disabled" or "decreased earning capacity" are a disadvantage. Although such fears are understandable they may cause problems at the work site. The employer is likely to notice the frequent visits to a physician (if the diabetic takes these examinations seriously) and hypoglycemia during work can hardly be disguised. We therefore believe that the diabetic should discuss his disease and possible complications with his employer and colleagues at work. They should know how to help him as, for example, in the case of hypoglycemia. They must understand that a diabetic must follow his meal plans carefully even during work.

let the employer know

Diabetes and Driving

Repeated instances of discrimination against the diabetic who drives are perhaps the most frequent and conspicuous of problems. However, diabetics do not present a general risk to traffic safety. But there is still cause for concern because certain situations may limit or restrict the driving ability of the diabetic. Such factors include complications of diabetes and side effects of treatment. Laws governing the driving of diabetics are established by state licensing authorities. The Federal government regulates interstate travel of trucks, trains and buses. Driving regulations differ from one state to the next, but most require that the diabetic inform the authorities about his disease when he makes his license application.

diabetics and driving

Diabetics who drive must be aware of the fact that a sudden onset of hypoglycemia could endanger him while driving and even cause an accident. Just like any healthy person, the diabetic may be prosecuted if he cannot prove that he took all preventive measures to avoid an accident. The following guidelines summarize the precautionary measures and all additional rules which the driving diabetic must be aware of and respect. The following guidelines apply to the diabetic who drives:

important
rules for
driving

- Sufficient quantities of carbohydrates easily digested and quickly effective (lump sugar or candy) must be readily available in the car. If there is a possibiliity that the diabetic may go into shock, then he should not begin driving.
- If there is the slightest indication that he may go into shock while driving, then he must immediately stop his car (even in a zone where it is not permitted to stop). He must then eat carbohydrates and wait until the state of shock passes.
- The diabetic should never inject more than his usual amount of insulin before driving and must be very conscientious in adhering to his usual injection schedule. Diabetics who must take oral hypoglycemic agents should also not deviate from their schedule.
- The diabetic should not eat less than the normal amount of carbohydrates before driving.
- If the diabetic plans to drive for a long period of time, then he should eat a small snack every hour and consume a certain amount of carbohydrates every two hours.
- If at all possible, the diabetic should avoid long periods of driving which disrupt his usual daily routine.
- For his own safety, the diabetic should respect speed limits at all times.
- The diabetic should not drink any alcohol before or during the time he drives.
- He should always have his identification card or some other indication of his condition with him.
- Once a year the diabetic should undergo medical examinations to test his general state of health and his driving capacity.

Vacationing and Traveling

any vacation
is possible

Diabetics are not restricted in their choice of vacation spots, because due preparation allows the diabetic to control his blood sugar level even while traveling and vacationing. It is actually unnecessary to say more if you have been reading this book from the beginning.

104

Many people today differentiate between vacations for relaxation and those for adventure. We simply advise that the vacation contain elements of both. However, most vacations entail a different type of or more physical exertion than everyday life does. As a consequence the diabetic must readjust his measures of treatment to the conditions of his vacation.

More often than not, diabetics engage in sports primarily during the summer and their vacations. As a result, the diabetic must readjust his diet and drug therapy to these new conditions. Of course, the normal schedule for meals and intake of meals must be strictly adhered to during these times. Although vacation is a way to escape the everyday chores, it should never be a vacation from the correct measures of treatment.

It may be particularly difficult to adhere to the established diet while on vacation because it is often difficult to anticipate the meals provided by hotels, restaurants and boarding houses. One should not rely simply on the advertisement of these establishments concerning their food. Instead, one should rely only on what is proper in one's own judgment. Certain organizations offer complete vacation plans for diabetics for which they guarantee proper nutrition. (The International Diabetes Federation and the American Diabetes Federation may be contacted for further information.)

The diabetic is confronted with a special problem when he can reach his vacation goal only by using an international flight and crossing time zones, thus shortening or prolonging his day. Insulin-dependent diabetics must adjust the insulin dose and number of injections to these changes. If the day is very much longer, then it may be necessary to inject an additional dose of insulin, while of course also consuming more meals.

Moreover, the diabetic should not be misled by the temptation of meals offered on board the plane which are usually rich in calories and often not suitable for the diabetic.

He should always take a carefully prepared travel kit for his medication with him on longer trips, and this kit should contain everything which he normally needs at home or might use in an emergency.

Suggestions for the travel kit containing medicine

what should
be taken
along

- Usual insulin
- Short-acting insulin
- Disposable syringes and needles
- Glucagon Glucose in ampules
- In the case of treatment with pills, oral hypoglycemic agents
- Sugar or another quickly effective carbohydrate
- A certain amount of snacks
- Diabetes identification card (also translated into other languages)
- Strip tests/test tablets for urinary sugar and acetone

Diabetes Identification Card

We have mentioned the risk of hypoglycemia so often that the need for the diabetic to always carry a diabetes identification card with him should by now be self-evident. This card, which may be obtained from the physician or local chapter of the American Diabetes Association, should yield information concerning the name and age, details about the individual diabetes control, diet plan, required type and amount of oral hypoglycemic agents, and required type and units of insulin. The patient should always up-date his card. If the patient plans to travel abroad, he should have the information translated into the languages of the countries he will travel through.

never leave
without iden-
tification card

The patient may prefer a bracelet or necklace to an identification card. By contacting the Medic-Alert Foundation International (Turlock, California 95380), the diabetic may obtain a bracelet engraved with pertinent information such as his name, type of diabetes and a telephone number where emergency medical information can be obtained.

Information Organizations

We believe that there is a constant need for information for the diabetic. As in so many other aspects of life, one can never learn enough about diabetes and should continue to seek the latest information. In addition to the teaching nurses and physicians the diabetic may contact for information, he may also join the American Diabetes Association and obtain a special journal for

up-to-date
information

laymen entitled "Forecast". This publication costs $12 per year and another called "Diabetes in the News" is available free of charge. The American Diabetes Association is very active and has established local chapters in almost all states. The national headquarters in New York (600 Fifth Avenue, New York, NY 10020) should be contacted for further information concerning affiliates near the patient's place of residence. The many activities of this organization include lectures, films and courses in cooking, plus camps for diabetic children. The American Diabetes Association, the Joslin Diabetes Foundation (One Joslin Place, Boston, Massachusetts 02215) or the Juvenile Diabetes Association (23 East 26 Street, New York, NY 10010) may be able to provide more detailed information concerning early recognition and preventive measures, as well as on insurance plans, tax deductions, employment and the driver's license for diabetics.

12. Juvenile-Onset Diabetes

There are about 1 million cases of juvenile-onset diabetes worldwide. Of the total diabetic population, about 4 to 5% are diagnosed as children. The National Health Survey estimates that 1 in 1000 under age 25 is diabetic. By comparison to the group of adult diabetics, this figure seems low.

what the parents should know

If you are the parent or a relative of a diabetic child and are reading this section for his benefit, then you should not expect information which is completely different than that which was presented in earlier chapters. Most of the material presented here has already been discussed in greater detail in previous sections of the book. However, since juvenile onset diabetes presents special problems because the child often reacts differently than the adult to metabolic disorder, he must be treated slightly differently.

Typical Diabetes with Insulin Deficiency

In almost all instances of childhood diabetes there is an absolute insulin deficiency. This is the classic form of diabetes but there is also another type which is now observed more frequently in children than ever before. This adult type of diabetes is found in very obese children who have overeaten for such a long time that the pancreas is overstrained. For the most part, these obese children must be treated in the same way as adults with this type of diabetes.

causes of the disease

Parents of diabetic children often question why it is their child that was affected, especially if neither one of them is diabetic and if there is no incidence of diabetes among relatives. Here it must be repeated that the disposition to develop diabetes is hereditary. If is often not possible to determine exactly how the onset of juvenile diabetes was precipitated.

It is known that general infections as in influenza, pneumonia and other diseases can precipitate the development of diabetes if there was a predisposition for it. Diabetes often appears in children and adolescents while they recover from an infection or immediately thereafter. Other factors which may precipitate the onset of diabetes are severe burning or injury.

How to recognize juvenile-onset diabetes

symptoms and complaints

The first symptoms are so conspicuous that it is nearly impossible to ignore the disease. The most important symptoms are tremendous thirst, increased fluid intake, increased urination, weight loss, resignation, fatigue and decreased performance. Small children who have stopped wetting their bed now do so because of the frequent need to urinate.

Other symptoms include indications of a metabolic disorder and diabetic coma if the onset of diabetes is dramatic, sudden, and not immediately recognized. Actually, it is not difficult to recognize diabetes in children once this possibility is realized. Symptoms which are negligible at first develop so quickly that it is almost impossible not to diagnose this disease. For this reason the diagnosis is usually made within a few days or weeks. Support for the diagnosis is given by evidence from urinary sugar and the elevated blood sugar level.

First treatment in a hospital

The newly diagnosed diabetic child should always receive his first treatment in a hospital. The first goal of treatment should be to quickly bring the blood sugar level under control. An immediate effort must be made to normalize the blood sugar values by injecting insulin and adhering to the appropriate diet. At the same time the parents and the child must be informed about the nature of diabetes and the possibilities for treatment, so that the child will learn as quickly as possible to treat himself and needs the parents' help only in the beginning.

After being discharged from the hospital, the diabetic child or adolescent should continue to be treated by a physician, pediatrician or in special outpatient care. Later admissions to the hospital should be avoided if possible. Should the diabetes be treated in the hospital only, then the control of the blood sugar level may be possible only under hospital conditions and not necessarily in the everyday life of the child. Treatment would then have to be readjusted completely to the daily routine of the child.

Long-term therapy

Older children and parents are prepared for the time following hospitalization during their stay in the hospital. At this time they learn to assume responsibility and act independently in the treatment and control of diabetes. The family doctor should be consulted when necessary and should be informed of the child's understanding and treatment of the disease.

children can give own injections

Both the parents and the diabetic child should be capable of injecting insulin. Often children who are only 4 to 6 years old are capable of performing the injection. Obviously, the parents and the child should be informed about proper nutrition and should be able to follow the diabetes diet. Finally, the diabetic child must learn to test his own urinary sugar (if necessary, with the help of his parents) and must be able to read the results in such a way that he can readjust his measures of treatment.

Insulin for the rest of life

All diabetic children and adolescents are insulin dependent for the entire lifetime. The guidelines discussed earlier for the supplies, storage of insulin and technique of injection apply to children as well as to adults. There are no differences in the types of insulin available for diabetic children and for adult diabetics.

The physician will base his decision concerning the kind of insulin and the number of units on the results of the blood sugar tests. The physician will also establish the length of the intervals between meals and the injection site. In doing so, he will make an attempt to incorporate the following goals of long-term treatment into the life of the child as early as possible:

goals of long-term therapy

- To attain the best possible balance of the metabolism with only a slight excretion of urinary sugar.
- To allow the child to grow and gain weight normally.
- To avoid blood vessel damage by controlling the blood sugar.
- To overcome the exceptional position and inevitable special demands made on the child by the diabetes.
- Not to allow the diabetes to interfere with the normal everyday life of the child as he attends school, chooses a career and makes friends.

Of course the proper quantity of insulin used is an insufficient measure by itself to control the blood sugar level. The level can be controlled only if it is possible to balance the units of insulin injected, proper nutrition, physical activity and frequent self-testing of the metabolism. The blood sugar level is controlled most easily if several injections can be made per day. This principle holds true for all insulin dependent diabetics, including the diabetic child. For this reason the parents should not insist on only one or two injections per day. The physician in charge will decide whether only one, two or more injections of insulin are necessary per day. If the usual pattern of eating is taken into account, then two injections per day are almost always necessary and three per day would be even better.

frequent injections are better

The time required for the insulin to take effect determines the length of time between the injection and the meal. A ten minute interval is best if rapid-acting types are used or if a mixture of rapid-acting insulin is added to the dose of an intermediate type. If, on the contrary, the child uses an intermediate insulin without additional rapid-acting insulin, then the interval should be 20 to 30 or more minutes long.

It is also important for the diabetic child to learn how to adjust the dose of insulin (but not the type of insulin) according to results of the self-testing of urinary sugar values.

Acquiring this ability requires special practice. Since the activities of a child tend to vary a great deal from one day to the next, the insulin dose (and of course the carbohydrate intake) must be readily changed in an elastic manner. No general guidelines can be provided for individual cases since the methods of treatment must be adapted to the individual requirements of each child. The physician in charge must always be consulted before the diabetic puts these measures into effect.

Diet for the Diabetic Child

the most important diet rule

Adherence to a diet plan suited to individual requirements is the most important measure of treatment in addition to the insulin injections for the treatment of both the diabetic child and the adult. The most important diet rule for the insulin dependent child and adolescent is to distribute the carbohydrates over many meals per day. Of course, children and adolescents should avoid pure sugar as should all other diabetics, and they must be careful not to gain weight. The diet must be healthy and well-balanced, and must include adequate amounts of carbohydrates, proteins, fats, vitamins and other nutrients.

Some parents consider the physical activity of a child to be a factor which interferes once the insulin treatment and proper nutrition have led to adequate control of blood sugar level. This belief is wrong because the physical activity of the child is important in the treatment to improve the utilization of sugar. Since it is often difficult to measure the amount of physical activity and is not always easy to anticipate it, the proper balance is difficult to find. One must know the measures of treatment in times of additional exertion.

exercise is a must

The best time for the child to participate in sports or to go out and play is after meals. At this time the risk of hypoglycemia is minimal. The diabetic child should be instructed on the nature of the first symptoms of hypoglycemia and the action which must be taken in this situation. He should always carry some sugar or candy with him.

Generally speaking, diabetic children should not be excluded from physical education classes or sports. Such exclusion could

111

make the child feel discriminated against and could make him feel like a second-rate person. Diabetic children interested in sports may participate in most sports clubs and organizations.

Self-testing of Urinary and Blood Sugar and Treatment Adjustment

The same principles and goals for self-testing of metabolism apply for the diabetic child and the insulin dependent older diabetic. The treatment must be adjusted to each individual case according to the results of frequently performed tests.

The diabetic child should use the Clinitest or Chemstrip G for frequent testing for urinary sugar. The physician will determine the details concerning the times and collection of urine. Consultation with the physician will indicate the action which must be taken from results of the urinary sugar examinations.

goal: balanced metabolic condition

Only if all the measures of treatment — insulin dose, proper nutrition, physical activity and control of metabolism — are balanced, checked and readjusted to changing requirements can the metabolism be regulated and severe metabolic problems prevented. Such regulation is absolutely essential. Usually the diabetic child will have to undergo medical examinations only once every 4 to 6 weeks. The diabetes must be regulated as closely as possible, not only on the day of medical examination, but also in the interval between examinations. In fact, the attempt to demonstrate good results on the day of examination is usually a sign that the diabetes is not completely under control during the interim period. Late sequelae can be prevented only by maintaining control over the blood sugar level.

Critical Phases in the Course of Diabetes

Distinct stages can be anticipated in the development of juvenile onset diabetes.

It is almost always necessary to gradually decrease the insulin dose during the first weeks following the beginning of the treatment. During this phase of remission, the required dose of insulin can become so low that it would seem unnecessary to inject any at all. However, all experienced diabetologists agree

temporary improvement

that the insulin injections should not be discontinued completely. One important reason is that the remission will last only a relatively short period of time, after which the injections must continue anyway.

The remission stage occurs in many diabetic children; the estimated figure ranges from 30% to 50%. The length of the stage during which only a small amount or none at all is required is variable in length since it may last a few months or one to two years. During this time it is not difficult to bring the blood sugar level under control. At this time, the parents and children should begin learning how to live with diabetes.

no false hopes

This remission stage can raise false hopes in the child or the parents. Wishful thinking leads the patient who need not inject insulin at this time to believe that he has been cured. The remission stage can never be interpreted as a cure because after a certain period of time the insulin dependence will become more severe.

The next stage in the course of juvenile onset diabetes is defined as "total diabetes," which usually develops after one to two years and is characterized by the permanently elevated requirement for insulin. In this stage the beta cells of the pancreas can no longer produce insulin. The insulin deficiency now becomes absolute and permanent.

puberty — a critical phase

A deterioration of the metabolic condition in the diabetic child usually cannot be avoided despite consistent treatment in the critical phase of puberty. During this time, the growth and development of the child probably causes numerous other hormones to be altered, thus increasing the need for insulin and subjecting the insulin requirement to great fluctuations. Other factors which make the metabolic condition of this stage extremely variable are the rapid growth, the strongly increased or variable food intake, as well as the emotional restlessness and caprice of youth at this time.

All teenagers require a great deal of understanding from their parents. The diabetic child must learn to cope with his disease in addition to all the other problems he may experience. The adolescent often acts negligently or rejects treatment, thus endangering the treatment.

Generally speaking, the metabolism is more stable once the diabetic has grown to adult size and weight, as well as sexual maturity. Toward the end of the growth period, the required number of calories decreases, as does the dose of insulin needed. These diabetics will gain weight if they do not adjust their diet to the fact that they are no longer growing. The food intake and insulin dose must be readjusted to the new situation.

Growth and Development of the Diabetic Child

The diabetic child is usually underweight only as long as the disease is developing and is first recognized. Since the disease initially causes the child to use more energy than normal, weight reduction is a typical sign of untreated diabetes. Diabetes does not interfere with the growth of the child if the blood sugar level is under control, and the food intake and insulin dose are well-balanced.

normal
growth
possible

The intelligence and talents of diabetic children are average. Diabetes does not interfere with intellectual development if the blood sugar level is well under control and maintained with proper treatment. Diabetic children easily compete with healthy children of the same age group in school. More harm than good is done to diabetic children who are overprotected or sheltered. Under no circumstances should diabetic children receive special treatment in school or in their family and social life.

Kindergarten — school — career

A pre-school diabetic child whose blood sugar level is under control can certainly attend kindergarten. The parents of the child must of course inform the kindergarten teacher about all the details relevant to the child's disease. Naturally, kindergarten teachers must know that the diabetic child must always eat a certain amount of food at predetermined times. Moreover, the kindergarten teacher should make sure that the child does not eat candy and should know that strenuous physical activity such as long walks or vigorous playing with other children could cause hypoglycemia. She ought to know that she is to give the child candy, a lump of sugar or a banana in this case.

no sweets

The parents should not allow a small diabetic child out of sight. If at all possible, the parents should bring the child to the kindergarten or nursery school and pick him up again.

Just like all other chidren, diabetic children should receive a broad education which may be particularly important for the diabetic later in life. Children who develop diabetes before attending school generally experience less difficulty later, as compared to children who develop the disease while attending school. Pre-school children with diabetes have a chance to adjust themselves to their disease before starting school. However, children who develop diabetes while already attending school must cope with readjustment and school simultaneously. Since the child will not be able to attend school for a while, he may receive poor grades temporarily. Parents and teachers should then be considerate of the readjustment which the child must endure.

The teachers must, of course, be informed that they have a diabetic child in class. They should know about hypoglycemia, how to treat it and how to prevent its development by carefully watching the child and taking the proper preventive measures.

Diabetic children should not be excluded from field trips or camps. They are capable of participating in such extracurricular activities and should not be made to feel ostracized at any time. The child, parents and teachers must know how to control the blood sugar level for all types of physical activity.

A young person with diabetes can choose almost any career. He should base his choice on his interests, talents and education. Certain jobs are better suited for diabetics than others because they fulfill certain prerequisites. A suitable job is one with a balanced amount of physical activity that permits a regular daily routine, offers the possibility to test urinary sugar and to care for the daily meal plan. Certain jobs are not recommended for diabetics.

Vacationing and trips

Diabetic children will certainly want to go on vacation with their parents. A vacation with the entire family is the best way to ensure proper treatment.

The family with a diabetic child may choose any vacation site they desire if they are prepared to deal with any problems which may arise in connection with diabetes, and are experienced in treating diabetes including the self-testing of urinary sugar. The self-testing must be performed with great care before going on vacation and at the end of vacation. During this time, the treatment must be adjusted to changes in the physical activity of the child which is usually greater at this time than at school.

camps for
diabetics

Older children who do not wish to vacation with their parents could go to a special camp for diabetics (for example the Elliot P. Joslin camp for boys at Charleton, Massachusetts and the Clara A. Barton birthplace camp for girls near North Oxford, Massachusetts.) Summer camps have many advantages. Not only can diabetic children enjoy their vacation with a large group of children of the same age, but they can also meet others who have diabetes and have learned to live with the problem. The camp may offer a special opportunity to control the blood sugar level. Lastly, the camp may relieve the parents from the daily and sometimes taxing burden of caring for children.

The diabetic child must not be forced to attend a camp, but instead should express his desire to participate. Concerned parents who visit their children at the camp should be aware that the blood sugar level is sometimes treated slightly differently at the camp than at home and that the results of the self-testing may not be as desired during the first days at the camp.

13. Will Diabetes be Curable in the Future?

Having read this book, you are aware of the methods and goals of diabetes treatment and from your daily life you know how to live with diabetes. Surely you have hoped at some point that the future would bring a cure for diabetes.

We know today that it will not be possible to cure diabetes in the near future. It is a hereditary disease which lasts a lifetime and must be treated during the entire lifetime. At best, obese diabetics can reduce their symptoms by reducing their weight. Although diabetics in a latent stage of the disease do not exhibit any clear symptoms of a metabolic disorder, they are not cured in the medical-scientific sense.

Even though there is no cure for diabetes, medical progress is being made in the treatment of diabetes. New methods are being developed or tried for the first time in practical situations. Experts work on these new possibilities and sometimes introduce them to the general public in special articles or broadcasts.

artificial pancreas

One hope for the future is the glucose sensor and glucose monitor which are complicated devices that allow the glucose content of the patient's blood to be checked continuously. The resulting measurements allow precise insulin requirements to be calculated with the aid of a computer. These devices would allow the patient to carefully regulate his blood sugar level within certain established limits. Much research is still necessary to make such devices available and economical for all diabetics.

Intensive research is being conducted on problems of transplanting the pancreas or insular cells from a healthy donor to a diabetic. Although perfect solutions have not been found in this area, research so far gives rise to hope.

insulin in the future

In recent times, efforts to develop better and purer types of insulin have been particularly promising. Successful attempts have been made to induce certain bacteria to produce human insulin by changing their genetic makeup. It may be possible in the future to develop human insulin from bacteria on a larger scale and thus not only to increase insulin reserves, but also to reduce the cases of insulin incompatibility. In the meantime, however, insulin must still be injected and it is very important to master the proper technique for injection.

The hopes of diabetics and their physicians — your and our hopes — are therefore not completely unfounded. Certainly progress will continue to be made. All new findings will bring us one step closer to realizing the most important goal of the treatment of diabetes: bringing the blood sugar level under control permanently and thus preventing blood vessel damage. This goal is the core of diabetes treatment even today. If you conscientiously undertake all treatment measures, then you will normalize the metabolic disturbance. Only if you apply the proper measures of treatment each day can you prevent the dangerous complications and consequences of diabetes.

Postscript for Physicians

Much general information on diabetes, its dangers and possible measures of treatment has been gained from the experience of physicians, general practitioners, diabetologists engaged in research and finally from diabetics themselves.

The discovery of insulin to treat diabetes was decisive in prolonging the life-expectancy of diabetics. Diabetics today no longer die from diabetes, from the actual metabolic disorder, but rather from the late sequelae of diabetes. The fate of the diabetic to be exposed to vascular damage clearly depends on the control the diabetic has over his blood sugar levels. Conclusive evidence gained in recent years from prospective studies, transplantations in diabetic animals, studies about pancreas and kidney transplantations in human beings, and large scale long-term studies shows the importance of bringing the blood sugar under control to prevent the development of late sequelae.

The two major points in the treatment of diabetes are therefore the following: one is the prevention of acute complications — since the discovery of insulin almost 60 years ago, the treatment of diabetes has permitted lives to be saved and the life-expectancy to be raised. The second major point is that vascular damage can be prevented or at least delayed if the blood sugar levels are brought under control permanently.

The results of the long-term studies are confirmed by the daily experience of treating diabetics. In our large outpatient clinic for diabetics we have found that it is not always easy to turn medical theory into general practice for the diabetic. We have realized how important it is to incorporate the process of informing, motivating and examining the diabetic into our treatment program. A patient can cooperate efficiently with his physician and prevent late sequelae only if he is well-informed and able to execute the treatment measures prescribed. The diabetic must become an expert in his own disease. In practical terms, this means that the diabetic must be able to plan and prepare his diet properly, must master the art of administering oral hypoglycemic agents, perform self-testing of urinary and blood sugar independently, and be able to adapt measures of treatment to changes in the metabolic condition.

We do not always have enough time available in our medical consultations to give the diabetic all the pertinent information, explain all the measures of successful treatment, or to instruct him in testing of his urinary and blood sugar. For this reason, we have chosen to write this book using our extensive experience with a large number of diabetics. This experience has helped us in our efforts to explain diabetes in a comprehensive and concise manner, and to motivate the diabetic to cooperate in the control and treatment of his disease. We do not claim to have found the perfect solution and do not deny that the book was influenced by personal experience. If you have any suggestions for improvement or would like to voice any other opinions, please write to the publishers.

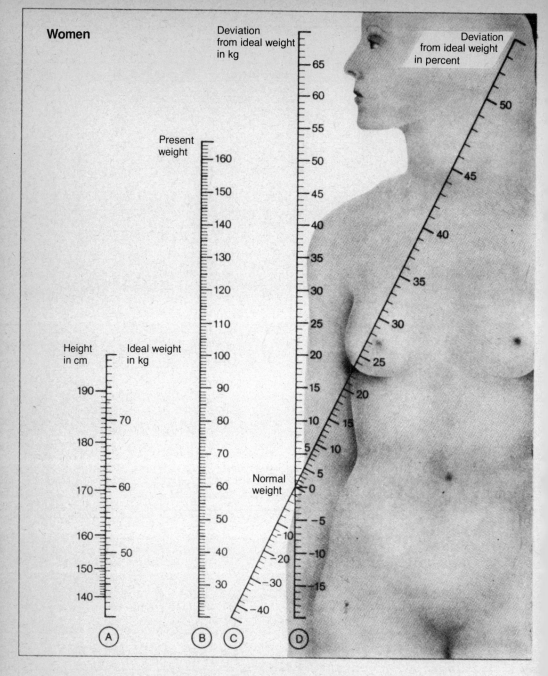

Women

Deviation from ideal weight in kg

Deviation from ideal weight in percent

Present weight

Height in cm

Ideal weight in kg

Normal weight

Ⓐ   Ⓑ   Ⓒ   Ⓓ

Normal weight: height in centimeters minus 100 = weight in Kilograms
Ideal weight for women: normal weight minus fifteen percent
Ideal weight for men: normal weight minus ten percent

This graph will show you what your ideal weight is, how much overweight (or underweight) you are in kg. and what percentage overweight (or underweight).

  1. Find your height on scale A (if you know your height only in inches, multiply the total inches by

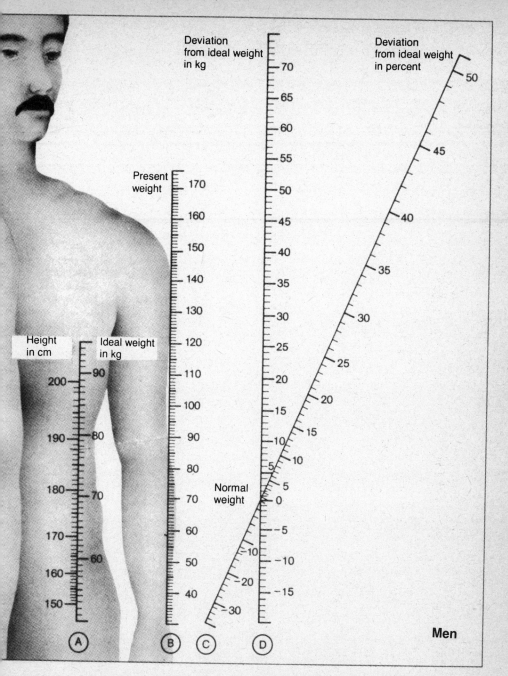

Deviation from ideal weight in kg

Deviation from ideal weight in percent

Present weight

Height in cm

Ideal weight in kg

Normal weight

Men

A

B

C

D

2.540). Put a dot on the vertical line. By looking on the righthand side of chart A you can now see what your ideal weight should be. (If you measure in pounds multiply the ideal weight on the chart by 2.205). 2. On chart B find your actual weight (multiply pounds by .4536). Put a dot on the vertical line. 3. With a straightedge draw a line between the dots on A and B and continue the line until it passes through C. The point at which the line insersects C and D tells you how many kg. (multiply by 2.205 = pounds) you are overweight and by what percentage.
  You are still *normal* weight if your present weight is 5% above or below the ideal weight.

Calculation chart for calorie expenditure (women)

1. Determine weight and height wearing light clothing and no shoes. (Kg = lbs. × .4536; cm = inches × 2.540)
2. Calculate the energy requirement, taking sex, physical activity, height and weight into account.

Women	Height	Energy requirement for ideal weight			Energy requirement for weight loss up to 20% overweight			Energy requirement for weight loss more than 20% overweight		
	cm.	kg.	Cal.	Joule	kg.	Cal.	Joule	kg.	Cal.	Joule
Light physical activity	150	43	2000	8360	52	1200	5020	60	1000	4180
	155	47	2000	8360	56	1200	5020	66	1000	4180
For example, teacher,	160	51	2100	8780	61	1300	5430	71	1000	4180
seamstress, secretary,	165	55	2100	8780	66	1300	5430	77	1000	4180
retired woman,	170	60	2200	9200	77	1400	5850	84	1000	4180
interpreter and	175	64	2200	9200	77	1400	5850	90	1000	4180
ticket saleswoman	180	68	2300	9610	82	1500	6270	95	1100	4600
	185	72	2300	9610	86	1500	6270	100	1100	4600
Average physical	150	43	2500	10450	52	1700	7110	60	1300	5430
activity	155	47	2500	10450	56	1700	7110	66	1300	5430
	160	51	2600	10870	61	1800	7520	71	1400	5850
For example, housewife,	165	55	2600	10870	66	1800	7520	77	1400	5850
cleaning woman, factory	170	60	2700	11290	72	1900	7940	84	1500	6270
worker, saleswoman,	175	64	2700	11290	77	1900	7940	90	1500	6270
waitress, nurse,	180	68	2800	11700	82	2000	8360	95	1600	6690
stewardess.	185	72	2800	11700	86	2000	8360	100	1600	6690
*Strenuous physical	150	43	3000	12540	52	2200	9200	60	2000	8360
activity	155	47	3000	12540	56	2200	9200	66	2000	8360
	160	51	3100	12960	61	2300	9610	71	2100	8780
For example, washing	165	55	3100	12960	66	2300	9610	77	2100	8780
clothes by hand, farmer's	170	60	3200	13380	72	2400	10030	84	2200	9200
wife, packer in factory	175	64	3200	13380	77	2400	10030	90	2200	9200
	180	68	3300	13800	82	2500	10450	95	2300	9610

*Strenuous physical activity: it must be determined whether the job actually falls into this category or whether less physical exertion is required due to increased mechanization, making it necessary to classify the job under medium physical activity.

Calculation chart for calorie expenditure (men)

Note: this energy requirement table is calculated for adults between ages 36 and 55. Adults between 19 and 35 need about 100 calories more (about 418 joules). Adults over 55 years of age need about 100 to 200 calories less (418 to 836 joules).

Men	Height	Energy requirement for ideal weight			Energy requirement for weight loss up to 20% overweight			Energy requirement for weight loss more than 20% overweight		
	cm.	kg.	Cal.	Joule	kg.	Cal.	Joule	kg.	Cal.	Joule
Light physical activity — **does not require physi-** **cal exertion** For example, teacher, civil servant, accountant, watchmaker.	155	50	2100	8780	60	1300	5430	70	1000	4180
	160	54	2200	9200	65	1400	5850	76	1000	4180
	165	59	2300	9610	70	1500	6270	82	1100	4600
	170	63	2400	10030	75	1600	6690	88	1200	5020
	175	68	2400	10030	81	1600	6690	95	1200	5020
	180	72	2400	10450	86	1700	7110	101	1300	5430
	185	77	2600	10870	92	1800	7520	108	1400	5850
	180	81	2700	11290	97	1800	7940	113	1500	6270
Average physical **activity** For example, carpenter, blacksmith, mechanic, weaver, physician, agent	155	50	2700	11290	60	1900	7940	70	1500	6270
	160	54	2800	11700	65	2000	8360	76	1600	6690
	165	59	2900	12120	70	2100	8780	82	1700	7110
	170	63	3000	12540	75	2200	9200	88	1800	7520
	175	68	3000	12540	81	2200	9200	95	1800	7520
	180	72	3100	12960	86	2300	9610	101	1900	7940
	185	77	3200	13380	92	2400	10030	108	2000	8360
	190	81	3300	13800	97	2500	10450	113	2100	8780
*Strenuous physical **activity** For example, butcher, bricklayer, construction worker, lumberjack, miner.	155	50	3300	13800	60	2500	10450	70	2100	8780
	160	54	3400	14210	65	2600	10870	76	2200	9200
	165	59	3500	14630	70	2700	11290	82	2300	9610
	170	63	3600	15050	75	2800	11700	88	2400	10030
	175	68	3600	15050	81	2800	11700	95	2400	10030
	180	72	3700	15470	86	2900	12110	101	2500	10450
	185	77	3800	15870	92	3000	12540	108	2600	10870
	190	81	3900	16290	97	3100	12960	113	2700	11290

Strenuous physical activity: it must be determined whether the job actually falls into this category or whether less physical exertion is required due to increased mechanization, making it necessary to classify the job under medium physical activity.

Substitute Foods List

The following lists indicate the carbohydrate, protein and fat content of each food and the calories it contains. This information helps the diabetic plan a nutritious and varied menu by making it possible to discover how much of one food may be substituted for another. The chapter on the diabetes diet should be consulted for more details.

Reminders
1. The portions specified in each list are interchangeable because they contain the same amounts of carbohydrates, protein and fat. For example, if your menu plan calls for one meat substitute, then you may substitute one egg, one ounce of cheese or two ounces of cottage cheese.
2. When you substitute one food for another in the same list, be careful to substitute the same quantity. For example, if your meal plan calls for two bread substitutes, then you may eat two slices of bread, or half a cup of corn plus half a cup potatoes, or one-third cup rice plus one slice of bread. In other words, one slice of bread equals one-third cup of rice or one-half cup of potato.
3. Consult the meal plan for 1000 calories outlined in the chapter on the diabetes diet for examples of food substitution.
4. For more information ask for an "exchange list for meal planning" from the American Diabetes Association, 600 Fifth Avenue, New York, New York 10020.

Note: certain vegetables are included in this list of bread exchanges because they contain a large quantity of carbohydrates. Each portion contains:
  carbohydrates: 12 grams
  calories: 70
Each portion is about equivalent to one slice (30 grams) bread.

Bread
rye, white, whole wheat — 1 slice
bagel — ½
biscuit — 1 (2 inch diameter)
(dry) bread crumbs — ¼ cup
corn bread — 2 inch square
english muffin — ½
hamburger roll — 2 ounces
hotdog roll — 1½ ounces
muffins (corn, bran, plain) — 1 small
  (2 inch diameter)
Cake
angel or sponge cake without icing —
  1½ inch cube
Cereal
dry — ¾ cup
cooked — ¾ cup
Crackers
graham — 2 (2½ inch squares)
melba toast — 5 thin slices
oyster — 20
pretzels (3-ring) — 6
pretzels (very thin sticks) — 65
Ritz — 7
Rye thins — 9
Saltines — 6
Triscuit — 5

Wheat thins — 12
Zwieback — 3

Flour
tapioca, corn starch, arrowroot — 2½ tsp
macaroni (noodles, shells, spaghetti) — ½ cup
matzo — 1 6-inch square
popcorn (unbuttered) — 1½ cup
rice — ⅓ cup
Vegetables
beans
  baked without molasses and brown
    sugar — ¼ cup
  shell (lima, kidney, lentil) — ⅓ cup
chestnuts — 5 large
water chestnuts — 12
corn — ⅓ cup or ½ medium ear
parsnips — ½ cup
peas (dried, or green cooked) — ½ cup
potatoes — ½ medium
whipped potatoes — ½ cup
sweet or yams (fresh) — ¼ cup
squash — ½ cup
sweet or yams (fresh) — ¼ cup
pumpkin — ¾ cup
squash, winter — ½ cup
tomato sauce — ¾ cup

Vegetable substitutes

Note: Vegetables can be divided to three different categories. The first category (section 1) includes those which may be used as desired. The second section includes the so-called three percent vegetables and the third section includes the so-called six percent vegetables. Please note that a one cup serving of a three percent vegetable is equal to a half cup serving of a six percent vegetable.

Section #1 (may be used as desired)

chinese cabbage
dill pickles
endive
lettuce
parsley
radishes
watercress

Section #2 Three percent vegetables

Serving size: *1 cup (150 grams)*
Nutritional value:
    5 grams carbohydrate
    2.5 grams protein
    calories: 25

asparagus
bean sprouts
broccoli
cabbage
cauliflower
celery
collard greens
cucumber
eggplant
green peppers
mushrooms
sauerkraut
spinach
squash, summer
string beans
turnips
zucchini

Section #3 Six percent vegetables

Serving size:
    ½ cup (75 grams)
Nutritional values:
    5 grams carbohydrate
    1.2 grams protein
    calories: 25

beans, green or yellow
beets
brussel sprouts
carrots
green peas
leeks
okra
onions
pumpkin
red peppers
squash, winter (boiled)
tomato
tomato sauce
vegetable juice

There are three kinds of fruit exchanges: section #1: small fruits; section #2: medium fruits; section #3: juices.

Section #1: Small fruits

Nutritional value:
10 grams carbohydrate
calories: 40

apricots, fresh — 2 medium
  dried — 4 halves
blackberries — ⅓ cup
blueberries — ½ cup
boysenberries — ½ cup
cherries — 10 large
figs, fresh — 1 large
  dried — 1 small
grapes — 12
lemon — 3 average
plums — 2 small
prunes (cooked) — 2 medium
raspberries — ½ cup
strawberries — 1 cup

Section #2: Medium fruits

Nutritional value:
15 grams carbohydrates
calories: 50

apples — 1 small
banana — ½ medium
cantaloupe — ¼ (6 inch dia.)
grapefruit — ½ small
honeydew melon — ⅛ (7 inch dia.)
nectarine — 1 small
orange — 1 small
peach — 1 medium
pear — 1 small
pineapple — ½ cup (3 slices)
tangerine — 2 small
watermelon — 1½ cup

Section #3: Juices

Nutritional value:
10 grams carbohydrate
calories: 40
Note: the diabetic should drink
  unsweetened jucies only.

apple juice or cider — ⅓ cup
grapefruit juice — ½ cup
orange juice — ½ cup
pineapple juice — ⅓ cup
prune juice — ¼ cup
also: apple juice with no sugar added — ½ cup
fruit cocktail with no sugar added — ½ cup
Avoid the following:
dates — 2
raisins — 2 tbsp

Meat substitutes

Nutritional value:
7 grams protein
5 grams fat
calories: 73

Cheese
cheddar, American — 1 ounce
Swiss — 1 ounce (1 slice)
cottage cheese — 2 ounces (¼ cup)
Egg — 1 medium
Fish
halibut, perch
  sole — 1 ounce
salmon, tuna — ¼ cup
sardines — 3 medium
shellfish
  clams, oyster
  scallop, shrimp — 5 small
crab, lobster — 1 ounce
Meat
beef — 1 ounce
ham — 1 ounce
lamb — 1 ounce
organ meats — 1 ounce
pork — 1 ounce
veal — 1 ounce
cold cuts — 1½ ounces
vienna sausages — 2
Poultry (fowl without skin) — 1½ ounces

Fat substitutes

Nutritional value:
5 grams fat
calories: 45

avocado — ⅛ whole (4 inch dia.)
bacon, crisp — 1 strip
butter — 1 tsp
cream
  half and half — 3 tbsp
  heavy, 40% — 1 tbsp
  light, 20% — 2 tbsp
  sour — 4 tsp
  whipped — 2 tsp
cream cheese — 2 tsp
salad dressing
  French — 1 tbsp
  Italian — 1 tbsp
  Roquefort — 2 tsp
lard — 1 tsp
margarine — 1 tsp
mayonnaise — 1 tsp
nuts (63 cal. and more)
  almonds — 5
  brazil — 1
  cashews — 5
  peanuts — 11
  walnuts — 4 halves
oil
  corn — 1 tsp
  olive — 1 tsp
  peanut — 1 tsp
  safflower — 1 tsp
olives
  black — 2 large
  green — 6 medium
peanut butter — 1 tsp

Milk and milk products substitutes

Nutritional value:
12 grams carbohydrate
8 grams protein
fats vary as shown in list below
calories: vary as shown below

Food	Portion	Fat	Cal
buttermilk	1 cup	none	80
evaporated			
skim	½ cup	none	80
whole	½ cup	10 grams	170
nonfat dry milk			
(powder)	⅓ cup	none	80
skim milk			
skim	1 cup	none	80
1% butterfat	1 cup	2.5 gm.	107
2% butterfat	1 cup	5 gm.	125
whole	1 cup	10 gm.	170
yogurt, plain			
made with skim	1 cup	5 gm.	125